PRESCRIPTION
FOR
PROTON RADIATION

PRESCRIPTION

FOR

PROTON RADIATION

REAL PATIENT STORIES, EXPERT PHYSICIAN INPUT ON A HIGHLY PRECISE FORM OF RADIATION THERAPY

DENISE DURGIN

NEW DEGREE PRESS
COPYRIGHT © 2021 DENISE DURGIN

PRESCRIPTION FOR PROTON RADIATION
Real Patient Stories, Expert Physician Input on a Highly Precise Form of Radiation Therapy

ISBN	978-1-63676-486-3	*Paperback*
	978-1-63730-395-5	*Kindle Ebook*
	978-1-63730-396-2	*Ebook*

To the patients and families, who need our stories to be told.

*To the physicians, nurses, radiation therapists and teams
who cared for us, fought for us and helped us heal.*

CONTENTS

———

INTRODUCTION

———

You have cancer. You know it's in your body. You need radiation treatment to kill it. Your doctor prescribes the radiation, but your health insurance won't authorize the treatment. It claims the treatment your doctor prescribes is medically unnecessary and authorizes another treatment plan, without meeting you or examining you. Imagine this happening over a few weeks or months, and your cancer treatment is delayed.

Stop imagining. This is happening in the United States to cancer patients seeking proton radiation treatment. A cancer treatment that's been approved by the FDA since 1988.

According to the American Society for Radiation Oncology (ASTRO), each week of delay in starting cancer therapy is linked to a 1.2 percent to 3.2 percent increased risk of death. So, while insurance is deciding whether to treat patients, patients are further stressed and potentially put at risk.

I know this is happening. It happened to me, and I fought back.

As my radiation oncologist, Michael J. Eblan MD, Radiation Oncology Associates, PC and Allison Scull, Referral Coordinator Manager at the Maryland Proton Treatment Center (MPTC), worked to get my treatments approved by UnitedHealthcare (UHC), almost eight weeks had passed since my mastectomy. Since cancer was found in my lymph node during the mastectomy, I needed radiation as no one knows where the cancer goes after it spreads to the lymph node!

Dr. Eblan and Allison were working on getting UHC to approve payment for proton radiation since April of 2018. As I moved into May, time was running out. I touched base with my oncologist, Kathleen K. Harnden, MD, to update her on the lack of insurance approval and to see whether I could start endocrine therapy, the next stage of treatment after radiation.

I'll never forget that phone call with Dr. Harnden.

"You need to be treated. You can't wait for insurance to approve it. Each week you wait for an approval, you increase your rate of recurrence of cancer in your body."

This both scared me and frustrated me. I felt backed into a corner by my insurance provider and the stress mounted.

I spoke to Dr. Eblan and he agreed with Dr. Harnden, so I decided to pay out of pocket. I thought I could use a few credit cards and get some travel points out of this pit stop with cancer. Dr. Eblan scheduled treatment to start on May 7, 2018 at MPTC.

On May 4, 2018, the same day I decided to pay out of pocket, hours later my case was overturned by UHC. I cried when Dr. Eblan called to tell me.

I thought:

How can this happen, we have insurance coverage?

Is this happening to other people?

If so, how can I help fix the problem of insurance delays, appeals, and denials?

How can I share my story that my case was overturned to provide hope for others?

During twenty-eight rounds of proton treatments, sitting on the radiation table and as I travelled to MPTC, an hour from my home, I thought about patients who didn't have resources or might not know about protons. I felt I knew these people even though I didn't. I started worrying about people I hadn't met.

I knew after I finished my treatments, I wanted to give back in some way and provide resources for patients to learn about proton radiation.

In June of 2018, I finished treatment and went from thinking about protons to action. I started to talk to healthcare providers and read more about insurance denials and appeals. Some patients had their cases overturned and insurance covered the treatment, some didn't.

I researched how often patients were being delayed treatments due to the insurance prior authorization process, which you'll learn about later in this book.

I set up a Google alert for "proton radiation." I launched my own website, www.protonradiationbuddy.com, which aims to provide information about proton radiation and share patient stories who've been treated with protons. Like Michelle, who shared her story of how she found proton radiation for an inoperable tumor that resided on her optic nerve. Michelle was treated at MPTC, and her treatments were approved by her insurance, without hassle, the way it should be.

By November of 2018, I received a Google alert with a startling headline—a major case was overturned! CNBC reported:

> *"A jury has ordered Aetna to pay more than $25 million to the family of an Oklahoma City woman who died a year after the insurance company refused to cover a type of radiation therapy."*

I thought: *Wow, there are people fighting back. I need to do more.*

In January of 2019, over brunch with my husband's nephew Brian and his wife Jenny, who are both physical therapists, I started talking about proton radiation and my experience with my insurance provider. Jenny said, "You need to meet my friend from college, Kate Weissman. This happened to her. It was stressful and insurance didn't pay for her treatment. She was on CNN news. I'm sure she'd like to tell you her story."

Jenny connected me to Kate. I listened to Kate's story in awe. You'll hear more about Kate's story later in the book.

Kate told me about the Alliance for Proton Therapy Access where she shared her story in an effort to help others. She encouraged me to share mine and connected me to Molly Daniels, the Executive Director at the Alliance. A few months later, I shared my story and became a volunteer patient advocate with the Alliance. On their website, there are patient stories who were first denied insurance coverage, but then the patient cases were overturned, and insurance covered their treatments. Like me, Janel Wright told her successful story with insurance coverage for her case on the Alliance website.

In February of 2021, Janel's doctors submitted her case for insurance to approve protons for a recurrence of breast cancer, this time on the left side.

"We appealed the first denial, and the staff at Seattle Cancer Care Alliance (SCCA) pulled together the terms of my insurance and the science proving the treatment's value. With this additional information, my insurer granted the second appeal."

Through my work at the Alliance, I met other cancer survivors who fought both their cancer and their insurance providers to cover proton radiation.

All the while, more overwhelming headlines were breaking into my inbox about proton treatment denials:

May 2019, from CNN: "Judge rips insurance company for immoral and barbaric cancer denials."

May 2019, from *The Boston Globe*: "An insurer denied her $95,000 cancer treatment, she's fighting back."

In the back of my mind, I knew our patient stories needed to be told to provide hope for others.

Meet my fellow fighters:

As Kim, twenty-five, a Doctor of Law in northern Texas, was fiddling with her wedding necklace at work, she noticed a lump in her neck. *Hmmm*, she thought. *Maybe I should get this checked out?*

Jim, fifty-seven, of Rochester, New York, didn't skip his annual physical and didn't worry a bit about the results he'd get. After all, he thought, he's healthy and exercises. He received his PSA as part of the routine exam. This year, things turned out different.

At twenty-seven, Keelin, a government relations professional, was sitting at work when she felt a lump on her neck. After a few days, she noticed it wasn't going away and was growing, so she decided to go to urgent care and get it checked out. After a referral to an ENT, her doctor told her she must have been sick, and her lymph node may be infected. It turned out that wasn't the case.

Kim, Keelin, and Jim were all diagnosed with cancer. Each needed a treatment plan. None were ***first*** prescribed proton radiation treatment, a specific type of radiation that more precisely targets the tumor and treated area, like a laser beam. Virtually no additional radiation is scattered throughout the body, unlike traditional photon radiation that passes through the body. Thus, protons protect healthy tissues and organs more effectively. If proton radiation is like a laser beam, think about photon radiation like a flashlight scattering additional radiation through the body, unknowingly hitting healthy tissues and organs, like the heart, lungs, spine, bowels, and brain. With photon, sometimes the healthy tissues and organs recover. Sometimes they don't.

At the time of diagnosis, Kim, Keelin, and Jim were confronted with three critical decisions regarding radiation treatment:

Should I stay with the recommended radiation treatment prescribed by my doctor?

Or is there another treatment that's going to preserve my quality of life and my body more safely?

Now that I've found proton radiation, will my insurance pay for it?

These are some of the many questions asked when patients find out they are diagnosed with cancer. They were the top three questions I faced when I found out I needed radiation. Yet, I didn't have friends I could talk to about proton radiation, and now I do.

This book can be read all the way through, and I hope you do. It can also be read by picking out specific sections that appeal to you.

If you're a cancer patient, or caregiver, learn from radiation oncologists and the chief medical officer of Varian, one of the manufacturers of the proton machine. Each have been interviewed specifically for this book. Each answered the same question:

What should a patient know about proton radiation?

In the pages that follow, you'll also hear from patients, physicians, advocacy leaders, attorneys, patient experience leaders, and others in the field of proton radiation with questions that you might be asking yourself right now:

What type of radiation am I receiving and why?

Why, in some cases, is this treatment option far superior to traditional photon radiation to preserve healthy tissues, organs, and quality of life?

What should I do if my insurance has declined to authorize my treatments on the first and second submission?

Should I advocate for myself? If so, how could I do it?

Receiving a cancer diagnosis is scary, and there are many options for treatment: surgery, chemotherapy, radiation, and endocrine therapies. This book will focus specifically on proton radiation treatment and help patients understand the physics of the proton dose, its precision, and how it minimizes damage to healthy tissues and nearby structures. Patients will also learn how to navigate the insurance approval process and learn about proton radiation from real patient stories.

The content shared in this book is written by me, a patient, and therefore isn't written to provide or substitute for medical advice.

I'm humbled to tell our patient stories as, ultimately, we want to share our experiences to help others.

As Cathleen McBurney, cancer survivor, proclaimed, "I'm telling everyone I know about proton radiation. It ultimately saved my life."

PART ONE:
EDUCATE

PROTON BOB

When I was first diagnosed with breast cancer, I was clueless. I'm healthy, work out, and eat a well-balanced diet. There's only one other person in my family that had cancer. Yet at fifty-two, the next thing I knew I had breast cancer. One of the funniest things my friend Heidi Day said when she learned I was diagnosed: "You eat all of those salads. You should've eaten the bacon." That gave me a good laugh. Nothing better than a laugh versus talking about my breast with friends and family. Ugh, that got so old.

After I learned about proton radiation and before I had my initial consultation, I wanted to know more about it. I had so many questions running through my mind. Even before being diagnosed with cancer, I liked to participate in my own health by being an informed patient, but I was told early on by my oncologist, Kathleen K. Harnden, MD, I should limit my research on the internet to only a few sites like breastcancer.org, the National Cancer Institute, and the American Cancer Society. Dr. Harnden's advice was so helpful to me. It kept me grounded. Although I felt like I was a bit of a nervous mess, I knew where to go to find evidence-based information. In other words, trusted information backed by science.

Yet there's still the human side to cancer. What did it feel like for other patients who had proton radiation?

I tried to find that answer and asked friends, family, and doctors I knew who were not part of my medical team. My friend Helen Kruger who I worked with at The Ritz-Carlton reached out to me, determined to help. She introduced me to her friend, Michael Long. He'd had proton radiation for brain cancer ten years ago and was doing so well! Talking to Michael before my treatments began was so comforting. He helped me prepare for what I could experience if I was prescribed this treatment.

I also reached out to the breastcancer.org patient forum and asked if anyone had been treated with proton radiation. Two patients responded. One was treated and eventually approved by insurance. One was prescribed protons and insurance declined it, so she opted for another treatment plan, and that's all I found.

Next, I thought maybe someone had written a book about being treated with proton radiation for breast cancer but there wasn't a resource. I kept looking.

Then I found Bob Marckini's book *You Can Beat Prostate Cancer: And You Don't Need Surgery To Do It*. Bob was treated with proton therapy for prostate cancer at Loma Linda University Cancer Center in 2000. He'd written a book about his experience and all the knowledge he'd gained over the years about prostate cancer, proton therapy, and all the other available treatment options for prostate cancer patients. In Bob's words:

> *"This is the book the author wishes had been available when he was diagnosed with cancer."*

Yes! This is how I felt. I wanted to know more about protons from a patient's perspective. I perused the book's content and was intrigued, so I quickly downloaded it onto my Kindle. Of course, I didn't have prostate cancer, but the book was about treatment options and Bob's journey finding proton radiation. Hearing his story made me feel safe and informed.

In Bob's book, he talks about his father who had prostate cancer and his brother Gene who was diagnosed with prostate cancer and treated in 1998 with radical prostatectomy surgery, which is the complete removal of the prostate and surrounding tissue. Seeing Gene in recovery had a profound impact on Bob. He hadn't been prepared for how serious surgery was and the debilitating after effects it would have on his brother.

After two biopsies, Bob started researching treatment options. He knew he wanted to avoid radical prostatectomy surgery due to the risks of surgery and the side effects that can greatly affect a man's quality of life, including the risk of impotence— roughly "50 to 85 percent" according to Bob's book.

After the biopsies were back and Bob was diagnosed with prostate cancer, his urologist said it was early stage and he recommended prostate surgery. Bob asked his urologist if there were other treatment options, and his doctor named two and neither were proton radiation. So, Bob asked his doctor about proton radiation instead of surgery. Bob's doctor said, in his book, "That's experimental. You could damage your rectum and wind up needing a colostomy."

Hearing this information devastated Bob, but he kept asking questions and kept researching. Bob ultimately decided on proton radiation for various reasons. In the fall of 2000, Loma Linda University Cancer Center was the only center in the United States that offered this treatment. Yet, his insurance approved his treatment, "100 percent no questions asked," according to his daughter Deb Hickey when I interviewed her and Bob for this book.

That's the way it should be!

When Bob and I spoke in the fall of 2020, he said he felt great, even all these years later!

After reading Bob's book, I learned a few lessons.

First, the book is well researched with facts, studies, and pictures that help a patient understand prostate cancer through learning about Bob's own diagnosis and decisions about treatment. Bob explains what the prostate is, "a walnut-sized gland located between the base of the penis and the bladder." He then explains the symptoms of prostate cancer (which many times are missed), the biopsy process, other tests, and then leads the reader down the journey to understand prostate cancer staging and options for treatment. He also makes the point that early detection for prostate cancer is vital just as it is for breast cancer and for any cancer for that matter.

Further in his book, I learned proton treatment isn't new—and it's certainly *not* experimental. It was approved for use in the United States by the FDA in 1988. It's been around for nearly sixty years and has gone through quite an evolution.

Looking back, my most impactful lesson in the book was how to advocate for myself and be part of the decision-making process *with* my doctors not *from* my doctors. It's nuanced but, essentially, Bob's message resonated that it's okay to ask the doctors questions. In fact, patients should, and Bob did!

By the time I started reading Bob's book, I had already had my mastectomy and reconstruction surgeries, so I saw first-hand what it was like when doctors worked together and reviewed my case to determine the best treatment option. I was also a couple of months into the cancer journey. I valued the doctor's advice, but I also didn't take a doctor's recommendation at face value. I found my voice and started asking a lot of questions, just as Bob discussed in his book. Luckily for me, my doctors included me in the decisions for my surgery and treatment options.

During Bob's treatments, he became friends with a few men who were also being treated at Loma Linda University Cancer Center. When their treatments ended, they talked about staying in touch and comparing notes. Bob volunteered to compile information and send a monthly email on how everyone was doing. This friendship and communication were the inspiration for Bob to start the Brotherhood of the

Balloon (BOB). What started in the year 2000 as a couple of emails to keep six guys connected after treatment turned into BOB, with over ten thousand proton therapy prostate cancer survivors.

BOB members represent all United States proton centers and several centers overseas. Members are from all fifty United States states and thirty-nine different countries. BOB has a comprehensive website—www.protonbob.com—full of helpful resources for prostate cancer patients, including more than one hundred former proton patient testimonials and "Life After Proton" short stories. You can also find FAQs about proton therapy, surveys, studies, and more.

After reading about proton therapy and Bob's experience, I wanted to find him, hug him, and thank him for his contribution. I haven't hugged him yet, but I've thanked Bob and his daughter Deb Hickey during our interview last fall.

Deb oversees the operations of BOB. According to Bob and Deb, the most important part of the membership—which is free—is their monthly newsletter. It includes the latest information on proton therapy and prostate cancer, as well as other valuable health articles.

I highly recommend Bob's book. He emphatically states in the introduction of his book he's not a medical doctor dispensing advice. As cancer survivors, we've both been through our unique diagnoses and treatments. We sincerely want to help people as a result of sharing our own experiences, education, and research we've found along the way.

When I asked Deb to explain why Bob published his book, she said:

> "When Bob was originally diagnosed with prostate cancer, he met with doctors of various specialties. Each one told Bob he was the 'poster boy' for the treatment option they specialized in. The more doctors he spoke with, the more confused he became, until he discovered proton therapy, which he learned was the single best treatment in the world for localized prostate cancer. Bob decided, after he was treated, to write the book that he wished had been available to him when he was diagnosed almost twenty-one years ago."

Bob and I had treatment eighteen years apart. Since then, Bob's published a second edition of his book. Yet there hasn't been a book published covering different disease types that were treated with proton radiation, so I decided to fill that gap.

Through our interview, I asked Bob the same question I asked the radiation oncologists:

What should a patient know about proton radiation?

In Bob's words:

> "The most important message in my book is about taking charge of your own health. Before making a treatment decision, do your homework. Don't just take your doctor's advice. Review all the options; speak with former patients representing each option you're considering."

Bob's right. Getting your homework done is vital.

Bob discussed other areas to consider when diagnosed with prostate cancer and the same advice can apply to many different types of cancer including breast cancer:

- "Get a second and third opinion."
- "Many times patients think radiation is radiation. Ask what type of radiation is prescribed and get familiar with the pros and cons of each."
- "Consider meeting with a doctor that can offer both proton and traditional photon radiation IMRT."

As Bob suggested to me, patients should feel comfortable asking questions so they fully understand the treatment options and the potential short- and long-term side effects associated with each.

Through writing this book I learned that in 2013 a close friend of Bob's and a BOB member, Chuck Kubicki, established the Robert J. Marckini Endowed Chair for Proton Research. Since its inception, the group has donated $13 million mostly for proton research and, according to Bob's second edition book, to date it's currently funded at $3 million.

I encourage anyone who has been diagnosed with prostate cancer to read Bob's book.

My heartfelt gratitude goes to Bob Marckini and Deb Hickey, who have paved the way and inspired me to make this book happen.

THE EVOLUTION OF RADIATION & PROTON THERAPY

———

"Those who received proton therapy experienced far fewer serious side effects than those who received traditional radiation, the researchers found. Within 90 days of starting treatment, 45 patients (12 percent) in the proton therapy group and 301 patients (28 percent) in the traditional radiation group experienced a severe side effect—that is, an effect severe enough to warrant hospitalization."

NATIONAL CANCER INSTITUTE, FEBRUARY 2020

The study from lead investigator Brian Baumann, MD, of the Washington University School of Medicine in St. Louis and the University of Pennsylvania, provides great hope for patients like me who've had proton radiation. Although patient survival rate was the same in the study, patients experiencing fewer side effects is meaningful to me. Others say the study had limitations, but Dr. Baumann noted:

"All patients in this study received high-quality treatment at a large academic medical center, regardless of whether it was proton or traditional radiation therapy, which suggests that the benefit of proton therapy that we saw is meaningful."

Looking back, radiation has come a long way since it was discovered in 1896. Decades later, researchers and scientists determined that radiation could cause cancer as well as cure it. According to the American Cancer Society, cancer risks from radiation was based early on from studies of the survivors of the atomic bombs in Nagasaki and Hiroshima. From these learnings and others, it was determined:

"The risk of cancer (from radiation) depends on a number of factors, the dose of radiation, the part of the body being treated, the age of the person getting it (younger people are generally at greater risk), and the use of other treatments such as chemotherapy."

According to the American Cancer Society, roughly 60 percent of cancer patients receive some form of radiation treatment as part of their care plan. Thankfully over the years, scientists continued to study and research the effects of radiation on patients' **nearby healthy tissues and organs**.

If a patient is prescribed any type of radiation by an oncologist, surgeon or other type of doctor, the referring doctor sends the patient to see a radiation oncologist. The radiation oncologist then determines the treatment plan. By the time I saw my radiation oncologist, Dr. Eblan, he was the fourth doctor on my medical team. The care team for cancer patients can evolve as the patient's case evolves.

Radiation is complex. Most people are familiar with the term, but many don't know what it means. So, I thought it would be helpful to provide a summary of the different types from research from the American Cancer Society, OncoLink, the National Cancer Institute, and my interview with Dr. Eblan.

Staring at the top, radiation can be delivered internally or externally.

External beam radiation means the radiation is sent to the body externally from a machine. There are different types of external beam radiation listed below.

Photon Beam Radiation:

- A type of radiation that uses X-rays that come from a machine called a linear accelerator (linac). The machine delivers the radiation dose at the surface of the body and goes into the tumor or treated area, **through the body and then exits the body. Therefore, healthy tissues and organs can be potentially exposed.**
- In certain cancer types, like prostate, breast, lymphoma, and head and neck cancers, depending on the treated area and number of treatments, photon radiation can cause "significant" side effects. Photon radiation is sometimes referred to as traditional radiation.
- Photon radiation has different delivery methods. Here's Dr. Eblan's summary.
    - **Two Dimensional** or 2D conventional X-ray therapy uses X-rays films to guide the treatment of photon beams to the treated area. This is an

earlier type of radiation that does not require advanced imaging or computerized technology and is most often used in an emergency to treat painful tumor metastases to the spine or brain.

- **Three Dimensional** or 3D conformal radiation utilizes advanced imaging, most commonly a CT scan to map and guide the radiation treatment. Many patients with breast cancer are treated with 3D conformal radiation, as the radiation fields can be angled to treat the breast but designed to block the heart and lungs, based on a patient's 3D anatomy from the CT scan.

- **Intensity modulated radiation therapy (IMRT)** is similar to 3D conformal radiation as it requires a CT mapping but uses multiple beams of photons spread out in many different directions. Each beam of radiation can be adjusted as it travels around the patient to more precisely target the intensity of radiation to the tumor or treatment area, while it uses sophisticated computer planning to minimize exposure of nearby structures—healthy tissues and organs. Most patients with prostate, head and neck, lung, and gastrointestinal cancers with complex shapes and sizes benefit from IMRT. IMRT often uses image-guidance radiotherapy, or IGRT, to improve the targeting of radiation and ensure protection of normal organs prior to treatment.

- **Stereotactic Radiation** According to Cyberknife. com this therapy is also known as radiosurgery, GammaKnife, CyberKnife, or stereotactic body radiation therapy (SBRT), and it delivers a very high dose of radiation to the tumor. Many different angles of radiation are used to converge a very high dose of radiation at a precisely targeted point in the body, like hundreds of flashlights all focused on one spot. It generally involves as little as one to five treatments because the dose of radiation delivered to the tumor is very high. It is used for certain patients and cancers like brain, liver, and lung, especially when surgery is not an option, because the high dose of radiation can be ablative to kill the entire tumor. It is generally not recommended when treating big tumors or larger target areas. The CyberKnife is the only radiation treatment that uses X-rays or photons with a robotic delivery system.

Proton Beam Radiation:

- This method more precisely targets the cancer cells through a proton beam moving at high speeds. It differs from photon radiation in that the proton beam targets the tumor or target area, but because of the physical properties of protons, the precise energy can be selected to stop the protons after hitting the tumor, so excess radiation **isn't** passed through the body potentially harming healthy tissue and organs.

Next, **internal radiation** delivers radiation into the body without using photons or protons.

Internal radiation means the radiation is treated internally to the body, not externally from a machine.

From the *Journal of Contemporary Brachytherapy.*

Brachytherapy:

- Sometimes referred to as internal radiation, where the radiation oncologist places encapsulated radioactive sources inside a patient to kill cancer cells requiring treatment. Because it's encapsulated, it's often referred to as "seeds." These seeds are roughly 4.5 mm in length and 0.8 mm in diameter. Sometimes these seeds are left in the body, sometimes they're temporary. This treatment is used in different cancer types like prostate, cervix, eye, and head and neck cancers. It's been used in prostate cancer for over thirty years.

In my interview with Dr. Eblan, I asked him to tell me more about the evolution of **protons** as a tool in the toolbox of radiation treatment options.

"With conventional two- or three-dimensional X-ray radiation, you could treat a pelvic tumor, the prostate for example, with a four-field box, but then every normal organ within that box would also be exposed to the full dose of radiation, which would include the bladder in front of and the rectum behind the prostate. In more recent years, intensity modulated photon radiation, or IMRT, has become the standard treatment for many cancers, including prostate, because it delivers more conformal radiation, focusing the full dose to the tumor while reducing the intensity of radiation to normal organs nearby such as bladder and rectum nearby. Many studies have shown IMRT to be superior to three-dimensional radiation. So thankfully we've come a long way since radiation was first discovered, as we now have many ways of delivering photons, or X-ray radiation, that are more precise and targeted to the tumor.

"Protons are the latest technology for targeting radiation more precisely. Radiation technology has evolved over decades to improve the delivery of a therapeutic dose to kill tumor cells, **but hopefully also limit any damage to normal tissue**. At first, a patient would sit or lay on a table while receiving treatment, and the tumor with all of the normal tissues within the radiation field would receive the prescribed dose. To promote recovery of the normal tissues, the treatment was fractionated, with the total therapeutic dose broken up into smaller doses that are given daily, up to several weeks.

"Protons are the next step in the technical evolution to more precisely target the radiation exactly where it needs to go, killing the tumor and further reducing radiation damage to adjacent organs, even eliminating any radiation exposure to nearby normal tissue."

—MICHAEL J. EBLAN, MD, RADIATION ONCOLOGIST,
RADIATION ONCOLOGY ASSOCIATES, PC

I've learned there are many reasons why one radiation treatment would be prescribed over another. Factors include disease type, location of the cancer in the body, recurrence of cancer (having cancer again), and a patient's health history.

When I heard I needed radiation, I didn't realize there were so many different types. Since I'm focusing on proton radiation and comparing it mostly with photon radiation, below is an excerpt from the magazine *Proton Therapy Today*. This resource does the good job of explaining the use of energy and how it impacts the body when comparing proton versus photon radiation:

> *"Before they reach the tumor, both radiation types have to make their way through the skin and surrounding tissues. The **photon**, with no mass and no charge, is highly penetrating and delivers a dose throughout any volume of tissue irradiated. However, most of the radiation is delivered only 0.5 to 3 cm from the patient's skin, depending on the energy it was initially given. It then gradually loses this energy until it reaches the target. As tumors are almost always in-depth located, the photon actively interacts with outer healthy cells and drops only a small remaining dose of ionizing radiation on the deeper diseased cells. Moreover, as photons are not all stopped by human tissue, they leave the patient's body and continue to emit radiation (exit dose).*

> *"On the contrary, the **proton** is a heavy and charged particle that gradually loses its speed as it interacts with human tissue. It is easily controlled and delivers its maximum dose at a precise depth, which is determined by the amount of energy it was given by the cyclotron (via acceleration), and can go as far as 32 cm. The proton is very fast when it enters the patient's body and deposits only a small dose on its way. The absorbed dose increases very gradually with greater depth and lower speed, suddenly rising to a peak when the proton is ultimately stopped. This is known as*

the Bragg peak. The behavior of the proton can be precisely determined, and the beam can be directed so the Bragg peak occurs exactly within the tumor site. Immediately after this burst of energy, the proton completely stops to irradiate. Proton therapy therefore allows to target tumors inside the body, precisely localize the radiation dosage, and spare the patient's healthy cells, offering a much less invasive alternative to treat cancer."

Translational Cancer Research provides an overview of the history of protons. For patients who were prescribed protons and told it was experimental, proton was first discovered by Ernest Rutherford in the 1900s. It was also discovered that charged particles (protons and light ions) have a finite range in matter which essentially means it has "stopping power" versus traditional X-rays:

"The fact that protons have a finite stopping power is one of the most distinct differences in proton versus photon energy."

Over the past hundred years, radiation therapy has evolved in three distinct ways: through technology, radiobiology (the biological effects of radiation at the cellular level), and clinical trials which will be discussed later in the book.

By 1930, American physicist Ernest O. Lawrence and his researchers had invented the cyclotron, which was used to accelerate proton to an energy high enough for cancer treatment applications. Then in 1946, a Harvard University physics professor wrote a paper on how protons could be used in cancer treatment. He cited the differences in "depth-dose, curve of proton and heavy charged particles" in comparison to X-rays (photons). He referenced the Bragg peak with the smaller amount of energy being released when entering the body and the largest amount of energy deposited at the tumor or targeted area, then the energy stops.

From the Loma Linda University Cancer Center website, patients can learn about the institution's history as one of the pioneers of proton radiation. By 1990, the first hospital-based proton facility was built in Loma Linda, California with a joint effort led by James Slater, MD, Loma Lina University Medical Center, and a government grant. Since then, Loma Linda University Cancer Center, known to most as Loma Linda, has treated 17,500 patients—more patients than any center in the world.

The second center opened at Massachusetts General Hospital (Mass General) in Boston, Massachusetts. According to their website, in 2001 the Francis H. Burr Proton Therapy Center opened there and has treated over ten thousand patients for both malignant and non-malignant tumors. In 2020, Mass General opened a second proton center, the Gordon-Browne Proton Therapy Center.

When I interviewed Carl Rossi, MD, Radiation Oncologist and Medical Director at the California Protons Cancer Therapy Center, he summed up the differences in proton vs photon radiation:

"The way that I describe it, our Pencil Beam system doesn't go all the way through the patients, which is what X-rays do. X-rays are great for doing diagnostic work, because they go all the way through the patient.

"At California Protons Cancer Therapy Center, we use the Pencil Beam system. I talk to patients and have them think of it as a 3D printer. I explain that we take the target and the computer breaks it up into a bunch of little millimeter boxes. And we paint the dose in the treated area layer by layer by layer. We're not spraying all around the treated area. A lot of folks have gone online, and they've looked at the various examples of how the Pencil Beam system works, how do the protons work, and they get it. They realize that we're just being more specific."

Photon therapy has grown in sophistication through intensity-modulated radiation therapy, or IMRT, which according to the Memorial Sloan Kettering Cancer Center uses advanced computer programs to calculate and deliver radiation directly to cancer cells from different angles. Cancer patients can receive higher, more effective doses of radiation while limiting damage to the healthy tissues and organs around it. Yet with IMRT, radiation is still passed through the body.

Similarly, proton therapy has also grown in sophistication and continues to evolve. As Dr. Rossi discussed in our interview Pencil Beam, scanning allows for the manipulation of the **beam** to create a pattern of protons to administer the dose more accurately to the unique shape of the tumor. When multiple scanning beams are used on patients, it's called IMPT.

But unlike IMRT, IMPT doesn't pass through the body or touch healthy tissue, structures and organs along the way.

In 2018 at the American Society for Radiation Oncology (ASTRO) annual meeting, lead researcher Steve J. Frank, MD, Associate Professor of Radiation Oncology, MD Anderson presented a study that found "the use of feeding tubes in oropharyngeal carcinoma (OPC) cancer patients treated with IMPT decreased by more than 50 percent compared to patients treated with IMRT. *This suggests that proton therapy may offer vital quality of life benefits for patients with tumors occurring at the back of the throat.*"

Dr. Frank's study and others that are in progress are evidence that proton therapy has so much promise for cancer patients. Yet, sometimes insurance declines payment, claiming it's experimental—but it's hard to imagine something that's been around this long is experimental.

As Dr. Rossi explains, the parallels of insurance denials and the use of the word experimental are constantly at play:

> *"Insurance denial is probably the most frustrating part of this whole process. Second, only perhaps to trying to talk with other radiation oncologists about why is it that your machine that supports X-rays is okay for the patient, but mine that doesn't do that is experimental."*

At the end of the day, proton radiation is both promising today and in the future. Clinical trials and research are important, and will give a sense of where we are in the field of proton radiation and where we're headed. Clinical trials and the future of protons will be covered later in the book.

WHAT SHOULD A PATIENT KNOW ABOUT PROTON RADIATION?

INTERVIEWS WITH NINE RADIATION ONCOLOGISTS

"Patients should know that proton radiation is a real and valid treatment. I think it still seems like it's a research project to people or not legitimate. But we can say with good confidence today that it is a legitimate radiation treatment."

—DAVID A. BUSH, MD, PROFESSOR OF RADIATION MEDICINE,
LOMA LINDA UNIVERSITY MEDICAL CENTER

Whew! When I first learned about proton radiation, I wish I'd seen this sentiment from Dr. Bush. Despite insurance denials claiming the treatment's experimental, it's comforting to know it isn't and, in many cases, it's medically necessary. I also thought it was important to lead with Dr. Bush's statement to lay the groundwork for the legitimacy of protons.

When I set out to write this book in the fall of 2020, my aim was to explain protons in layman's terms using analogies that people can relate to.

Let's start with the basics:

- **What should a patient know about proton radiation?**
- **Is it right for me?**
- **How do I know it is right for me versus a different type of radiation?**

I interviewed eight radiation oncologists from six different proton centers across the United States and in Canada. I also interview the chief medical officer, who is also a radiation oncologist, at Varian, a company that specializes in the manufacturing of proton machines.

I asked the same question to fifteen patients, who received proton radiation for nine different disease types. Patients weighed in from proton centers where they were treated like, Loma Linda University, Rutgers Cancer Center, Cincinnati Children's Hospital, Massachusetts General Hospital, Provision Cares Proton Therapy Knoxville, and MD Anderson Cancer Center.

So, starting with the group of esteemed radiation oncologists, I asked: **"What should a patient know about proton radiation?"**

> *"Let's start with what proton is and isn't. There are a lot of patients who have this idea it's not radiation, they'll come in and say, 'I don't want radiation treatment, but I want protons.' So I try to make sure I make it clear to them that this is a type of radiation therapy, in particular a type of external beam radiation, which is similar in that regard to photon therapy (X-rays) in that the machines are both outside the body.*

"But I'll illustrate the difference by talking about the physics and that we use the superior physics of protons, the fact that they come to a stop at some point in space, to reduce toxicity, and that in virtually all patients that we treat with protons, and we treat essentially all the things treated with photon therapy (X-rays), we're using it not because we get a better cure rate. There are a few situations where that's true. But by and large, it's not.

We're using it to get the same chance of cure with fewer side effects.

"I like to make sure that the patients realize that this is based upon science, and it's based upon physics, and it was something which was discovered in 1904—so very shortly after X-rays were discovered—and that it was also first proposed as a cancer treatment in 1946. Robert Wilson wrote his first paper on it. It was first used in 1954. So, there are a lot of patients who also will come in saying, 'Oh, my doctor told me it's too new. It's investigational. There's no background.' I'll say to them, we started this in the Eisenhower administration, do you think that's not enough time to understand how it works?

"I also want to make sure that people understand it's a type of external beam radiation which has superior physical characteristics. We've wanted to do this for a long time to take advantage of the superior physics. It's really been the last thirty years that we've been able to do this on

somewhat of a large scale and that continues, of course, to improve."

—CARL ROSSI, MD, RADIATION ONCOLOGIST, MEDICAL
DIRECTOR, CALIFORNIA PROTONS CANCER THERAPY CENTER

"The main point that patients should know about proton radiation therapy is that, first of all, proton therapy is not a magic bullet. With proton therapy, we're not necessarily conferring in most cases, a different effect on the cancer than we would with photon therapy or brachytherapy.

*"From a cancer management perspective, that's not where the value proposition of proton therapy is, it's really in mit-igating the toxicity of the treatment as it relates to the **spar-ing of normal tissues from unnecessary radiation dose, mitigating both acute and chronic toxicity of treatment.***

"Patients will often say, 'I need protons, because that's what's going to cure me.' What I would say is that, in most cases, photons are also likely to confer cure. But the value proposition with proton therapy is the conferral of a better toxicity profile in addition to cancer control. Some-times it's hard for patients to understand that, especially early in their patient journey, when really what's on top of their mind is how to beat their cancer. Proton therapy gives patients the opportunity to balance this with the pros-pect of a better quality of life after the cancer treatment has ended."

—GOPAL K. BAJAJ, MD, MBA RADIATION ONCOLOGIST;
PRESIDENT, RADIATION ONCOLOGY ASSOCIATES,
PC; VICE CHAIR OF THE GOVERNMENT RELATIONS
COUNCIL FOR THE ASTRO BOARD OF DIRECTORS

44 · PRESCRIPTION FOR PROTON RADIATION

"Protons are a very important tool to have in the radiation oncology toolbox. Protons, like photon (X-ray) therapy, [are] a form of radiation treatment that is externally delivered. The difference between the two techniques lies in the unique physical property of protons, which is that they lack exit dose past the point of the tumor that is being targeted. This allows protons to deliver less unnecessary dose to normal organs surrounding the intended target in comparison to photon (X-ray) therapy. Therefore, proton therapy can provide the opportunity to achieve comparable tumor control with a lower risk of short- and long-term side effects.

"It must be emphasized that there are instances in which proton therapy is preferred to photon therapy (X-rays), as well as situations in which the two technologies are equivalent. When deciding between the two techniques for a patient, there are many elements that must be accounted for in the decision-making process, such as:

'What is the specific tumor type we are treating?'

'What is the age of the patient?'

'What is the stage of the tumor?'

'Where is the location of the target relative to surrounding normal organs?'

'Has the patient had prior radiation therapy?'

'How far does the patient live from a proton center?'

'Can the patient afford to be away from work, family, and do they have transportation and housing means near a center?' (Proton therapy is a regional resource that is not available everywhere.)

"As such, we as radiation oncologists must educate patients and use this excellent tool in the most appropriate situations."

—ARPIT CHHABRA, MD, RADIATION ONCOLOGIST, DIRECTOR OF EDUCATION, NEW YORK PROTON CENTER

"I meet patients whom I believe would benefit from protons and I also meet patients that I don't think protons would be beneficial, and I think the key thing to remember is:

"Protons don't increase the rate of tumor control. It does not improve survival in that sense."

"That's something that I tell everyone because some public resources, such as proton center websites, are written in such a way that one can construe that. And as a person who really believes in proton therapy and wants to bring it to Canada, I'm very upfront that the rate of tumor control is the same between the two modalities (photons and protons). The only potential benefit that we can be sure about would be the reduction in late toxicities, which is paramount in kids and highly functional adults."

—DEREK TSANG, MD, RADIATION ONCOLOGIST AT THE PRINCESS MARGARET CANCER CENTRE IN TORONTO, CANADA

"Patients should know that proton therapy is the latest technology in radiation delivery, but it's not necessarily the right treatment for every patient with cancer.

"But protons are a treatment modality that needs to be part of the conversation for many types of cancers and many diagnoses."

"Protons can offer a safer method of delivering radiation to the tumor while minimizing the potential for collateral damage to the normal tissues and organs that are adjacent to where you need to treat. Often, we are able to spare the normal tissues adequately with the latest photon (X-ray), radiation technology. But in situations where conventional radiation (photons) may risk irreparable harm to adjacent critical organs such as the heart, liver, or spinal cord, protons offer the hope of safer treatment without comprising the radiation dose to the tumor and risking the chance of cure."

—MICHAEL J EBLAN MD, RADIATION ONCOLOGIST,
RADIATION ONCOLOGY ASSOCIATES, PC

"I get asked a lot of the same questions about proton therapy from inquiring patients. Patients ask: 'How is the dose different with proton therapy? Does it shrink the tumor differently and is it as effective?'

"Proton therapy delivers essentially the same dose and should confer at least the same level of efficacy in terms of cancer control as would be seen with photons. While the issue is somewhat complex, the primary reason one might consider proton therapy over photon therapy is the potential to spare normal tissues from unnecessary radiation dose, and therefore toxicity, which can be a considerable difference in some, but not all, clinical scenarios.

"When considering proton therapy, it is important to keep in mind that not all proton therapy is created equal.

The early generations of proton therapy, namely, passive scattering proton therapy and uniform scanning proton therapy, were not as precise or advanced as the more modern proton technology that is available in newer proton centers. That said, we owe much to these early centers and the experience gained using those technologies, as [they] helped the field advance to the level at which it is now. In the most current generation of proton therapy, pencil beam scanning proton therapy, we are able to use intensity modulated proton therapy (IMPT), to much more precisely and accurately target and deposit the radiation dose, which harnesses the inherent stopping power of the proton particle further and enhances the ability of proton therapy to spare normal tissues.

"In addition, some of the most recently developed treatment sites such as Emory University and the New York Proton Center have on board cone beam CT imaging, which allows us to be even more accurate in our daily setups. This allows us to be more confident in our ability to treat challenging tumors with inherent complexities such as thoracic and gastrointestinal (GI) tumors, where visualization of the soft tissue is critical to ensure accurate targeting of the treatment volume and historical setups using bone landmarks alone would not suffice. Very few proton centers to date have that technology, although with increased realization of the importance of this technology, newer centers are frequently including it in their development plans. Therefore, keeping these and many other nuanced subjects in mind is something for patients to consider when looking at their treatment options.

"Proton therapy is a more costly treatment compared with traditional radiation therapy. And the reason for that is simply because the proton particle requires a much heavier and larger machine to deliver it accurately and precisely, compared with traditional radiations photon therapy particle. The proton particle's charge is much, much larger compared with a traditional photon particle. So, because of that upfront cost disparity between protons and photons, we have found that it is much more difficult to provide access to proton therapy for patients due to some insurance barriers. And that's one of the areas that's concerning."

—J. ISABELLE CHOI, MD, RADIATION ONCOLOGIST,
CLINICAL DIRECTOR AND DIRECTOR OF
RESEARCH, NEW YORK PROTON CENTER

"Patients should be evaluated by a physician who has experience with both proton as well as photon radiation. It is estimated that about 20 percent of patients who currently receive radiation therapy would benefit from proton therapy.

"From my own personal experience when I was a radiation oncologist in Philadelphia (without experience with protons), I did not have that firsthand knowledge about protons, making it very difficult for me to determine who would (and would not) benefit from protons compared to photons. Now, after having firsthand knowledge with protons in addition to photons, I can have a detailed conversation with patients about the relative risks and benefits of protons compared to photons for each patient's specific case. It is also important for patients to know that while we have learned a lot about protons over the past few decades, there are some scenarios where we are still trying to determine how protons compare to regular radiation therapy. In these situations, it would be beneficial for patients to ask about opportunities to participate in clinical trials.

"I hear a lot of patients who are told that they are not candidates for proton radiation, and they cannot get radiation therapy. They're often told this by their medical oncologist, their surgeon, or radiation oncologist. Some patients research on their own and find a proton center. But it really should be that their providers and physicians are guiding them and telling them, 'hey, there might be this option that's there for them.' I think any patient who is told that they're no longer a candidate for radiation therapy, shouldn't necessarily take that's as it's written in stone. Things are changing and changing quickly. Patients could think about getting a second, third, or fourth opinion from an academic center that has all the latest radiation tools."

—MARK V. MISHRA, MD, RADIATION ONCOLOGIST,
ASSOCIATE PROFESSOR OF RADIATION ONCOLOGY AND
DIRECTOR OF RADIATION ONCOLOGY CLINICAL RESEARCH,
UNIVERSITY OF MARYLAND SCHOOL OF MEDICINE

"At Loma Linda we were involved early in the course. So, I remember those days, it didn't seem normal to have this treatment option. But, nowadays, it is normal for a lot of different disease sites, and, of course, a lot more available than it used to be back in the day. I think there's good evidence today, clinical evidence that it's beneficial in a number of disease sites. So, patients can feel more confident in receiving proton therapy for the indications that we have today, and that there's a lot of research going on for new applications going forward."

—DAVID A. BUSH, MD, PROFESSOR OF RADIATION MEDICINE,
LOMA LINDA UNIVERSITY MEDICAL CENTER

"Proton therapy represents arguably one of the most technologically advanced medical devices.

"Protons have the ability to substantially reduce side effects compared to traditional radiation therapy devices.

"The main differentiating features are that with standard radiation devices, the beam comes into the body and passes all the way through the body, irradiating everything in its path. With protons, the beam goes into the tumor to a predefined depth but doesn't exit through the normal tissue, hence reducing side effects."

—DEEPAK "DEE" KHUNTIA, MD,
SENIOR VICE PRESIDENT, CHIEF MEDICAL OFFICER, VARIAN

It was wonderful to interview all of the physicians and learn more about proton radiation. I was a patient who benefited from the Varian ProBeam machine when I was treated at the Maryland Proton Treatment Center. The ProBeam is so precise and, because of its pencil beam scanning abilities, it was able to cover my entire treatment area. Specifically, ProBeam works like a 3D printer, painting in the targeted area, just as Dr. Rossi mentioned.

The key takeaways for patients:

- Proton radiation isn't experimental.
- Not all proton therapy is created equal. Ask what type of proton radiation the center offers. In my case, I received treatment from the Varian machine which has pencil beam scanning.
- Consider meeting with a physician that offers proton and other types of radiation therapy.
- Some patients find proton therapy through their own thorough research, but that doesn't mean a patient shouldn't ask about proton radiation if it wasn't originally prescribed. Later in the book, many of the patients I interviewed found protons on their own, the way I did.
- Protons can substantially reduce side effects compared to photons.
- Proton therapy can be more costly, but not always. At the Maryland Proton Treatment Center, my treatments cost the same whether I had proton or photon radiation. It's best to ask at the treatment center before ruling it out that it's going to be more expensive.

I recently reached out to a breast cancer support group on Facebook. I asked the moderator of the site if I could post something about my book on proton radiation. I thought it might be a good idea to let patients know my book was almost ready for publishing and maybe it would help some of the patients.

She regrettably said, "no." She felt that proton is too expensive, and it would look like we were promoting it. I understood her point, but was disappointed as the whole purpose and inspiration for my book is to educate patients (not prescribe). Sometimes proton radiation can be more expensive, but sometimes it's not. This book is about so much more than educating patients about the cost. Until this conversation about proton radiation becomes more mainstream, I will continue to advocate.

My heartfelt gratitude goes out to all the physicians who helped create this chapter. I hope you, the reader, find their thoughts and advice useful. I know I did!

ACCESS TO PROTON THERAPY

___

"There should be no physician bias. Just because a physician doesn't have access to proton radiation at their own medical facility, it should still be offered if the physician believes the patient will benefit from the treatment."

—GOPAL K. BAJAJ, MD, MBA, RADIATION ONCOLOGIST;
PRESIDENT, RADIATION ONCOLOGY ASSOCIATES, PC;
VICE CHAIR OF THE GOVERNMENT RELATIONS
COUNCIL FOR THE ASTRO BOARD OF DIRECTORS

I learned through my own experience and from interviewing the radiation oncologists for this book, protons aren't right for every patient. But every patient has the right to know protons exist. I'm not dispensing medical advice. Rather, I'm encouraging patients to participate in their own care by advocating for themselves, so that access to different treatment options like protons can be discussed. This was hard for many people I interviewed, including me.

Further into my interview with Mark V. Mishra, MD, Radiation Oncologist, Associate Professor of Radiation Oncology and Director of Radiation Oncology Clinical Research, University of Maryland School of Medicine I asked him how patients could access protons:

> *"I think the most important thing is to be able to go and be seen by a provider who can talk to you about the benefits and the risks of radiation therapy delivered with the different types of radiation therapy that are out there."*

I agree.

When I was diagnosed with stage IIB ductal carcinoma in situ (DCIS) breast cancer in January of 2018, my husband Patrick and I were tossed into the cancer space searching for answers, yet many times we didn't know the right questions to ask. Consequently, I stumbled upon proton radiation in the strangest way.

Unexpectedly after surgery, I found out I needed radiation therapy, as the cancer ended up spreading to my lymph node and broke through it which means the cancer was invasive. In another blink of an eye, my diagnosis changed to invasive ductal carcinoma, IDC, stage IIB.

My husband called his friends to tell them he would miss their annual golf trip to Kiawah Island. It was their twenty-sixth year, and my husband told his friend Tim Hill he wanted to take me to radiation treatments, and he would miss the trip. By the end of the call, Patrick said to me:

*"I learned about radiation treatments, something called **proton** radiation versus **photon**. What type of radiation are you getting?"*

I said, "I have no idea."

Tim told Patrick that their fellow golfer, Jason Pappas, was the interim CEO at Maryland Proton Treatment Center (MPTC). Tim thought Patrick should talk to Jason. Patrick and Jason spoke, and later that day Jason made an introduction to Dr. Eblan and Dr. Chhabra.

Within a few days we had a consultation with Dr. Eblan.

I live in northern Virginia close to Washington, DC. At that time, I had three options for treatment. The first was the Maryland Proton Treatment Center in Baltimore Maryland, a hundred mile ride round trip. Then there was the Hampton University Proton Center in Norfolk Virginia which was 350 miles round trip from our home, or Georgetown University Proton Center about eight miles from our home.

Patrick and I researched all three centers, but we knew, because of the relationship we formed with Dr. Eblan after our first consult, being in his care was the best decision for me. In the end it was an easy decision but would mean a total of twenty-eight round trips to Baltimore. It was totally worth it.

Over the course of my treatments and 2,800 miles of travel, I had lot of time to think about plenty of things. Although receiving cancer treatments can create anxiety, and it certainly did for me, I remained rooted in a sense of gratefulness. I wasn't experiencing cancer treatments alone, and my husband and I could take time off work and could travel to receive treatment.

While spending time in the patient waiting room for treatments, I met other cancer patients—some had travelled from out of state, some from overseas. With all the time in the waiting room, patients built friendships with fellow patients and families. Adorned in my patient gown along with my fellow patients, I liked seeing familiar faces, smiles, and hearing conversations each day I arrived at the center. I especially loved hearing the cheers from patients who rang the Hope Bell, which is an event that occurs at the conclusion of radiation treatment in most cancer centers.

As I waited for treatments and at night as I laid in bed, I wondered what happened to patients who needed proton radiation but couldn't get access. With such a small amount of proton radiation centers in the country and in the world, who's getting access to this treatment?

Despite the reliance on their doctor's advice, some of the patients I interviewed for this book found out about protons from a second opinion, researching on Google, or talking to a friend like in my case.

In the University of Maryland Medical Center's (UMMC) video series, they featured five-year-old Phoebe Melling who travelled over ten thousand miles from Melbourne, Australia to Baltimore, Maryland so she could be treated at MPTC. Phoebe had a rare form of cancer in her sinuses.

Travelling from Melbourne to Baltimore for cancer treatments is courageous, and this can be a challenge with proton radiation treatment as Dr. Chhabra described earlier in this book. Once a patient is prescribed protons, the next step is figuring out where to go, and from there, is it even feasible to travel to the center? Ten thousand miles is a long way to go for treatment.

In my interview with Jennifer Maggiore, the Executive Director of the National Association for Proton Therapy (NAPT), she said:

"Seventy percent of patients in the United States travel more than one hundred miles for proton radiation treatments."

That's because, at the time of publishing, there are thirty-seven operating proton radiation centers in the United States.

There are only seventy operating proton centers around the world.

Many of the patients I interviewed for this book travelled across states, from North Carolina to Maryland, South Carolina to Tennessee and more.

It's 2021, and there are three proton centers now open within ten miles of where I live in Northern Virginia. But outside of the Washington, DC area, not only are there geographic challenges, but there's socioeconomic challenges, too.

When I was in treatment, I met so many prostate patients being treated with protons. I wondered if these patients were approved by insurance more often than breast cancer patients? I thought, 'could breast cancer also be a barrier to accessing proton treatments?

I wanted to find evidence this wasn't the case. I read a study in the *International Journal of Radiation Oncology, Biology, Physics* whose purpose was to report on healthcare disparities and inequities for prostate cancer patients accessing radiation therapy (RT). I thought I might find at least some of the answers there.

The study's initial query looked at 281 studies with seventy-nine meeting the author's inclusion criteria. After evaluating twenty-six years of literature and studies from 1991 to 2017, themes of inequities emerged in radiation modality type, including photon intensity-modulated RT (IMRT), proton therapy, brachytherapy, and stereotactic body RT (SBRT) in forty-three studies. The most common health inequities reported were age (twenty-three studies), race and ethnicity (sixty), socioeconomic status (twenty-two), insurance status (eighteen), and hospital or practice characteristics (twenty-four). The authors Katipally, Rohan BS and Curtiland Deville Jr., MD, concluded:

> *"Significant inequities in the utilization of radiation therapy (RT) for Prostate Cancer (PCa) exist, with the most published RT outcomes pertaining to age, race, socioeconomic status, insurance status, and practice setting. These inequities likely contribute to disparities in overall PCa morbidity and mortality."*

Another study, "A Population-Based Assessment of Proton Beam Therapy Utilization in California" by Arti Parikh-Patel et al. sought to *evaluate the patterns and determinants of proton therapy* in the state of California. The study design involved patients of all cancer types from 2003 to 2016, inclusive of those who had any type of radiation therapy and were identified in the California Cancer Registry.

Of the 2,499,510 people with a cancer diagnosis during this timeframe, 23 percent received some type of radiation therapy, and of that subset of 578,632 people, 1.5 percent—or 8,609 people—received proton beam therapy. Proton therapy was most often used in prostate cancer (41.3 percent), breast (14 percent), eye (11.7 percent), lung (6.1 percent), and brain (6 percent). In conclusion:

> *"Significant differences exist in proton therapy use by demographics and health insurance type. The identified racial and socioeconomic disparities merit further investigation."*

Some of the key takeaways from this study were:

- The Medicare patients who were covered were more likely to receive proton beam therapy compared with patients with private insurance.
- Compared with non-Hispanic whites, all other racial/ethnic groups had significantly lower odds of being treated with proton beam therapy, across various cancer types, after accounting for other relevant demographic and clinical factors.

I wasn't naïve to the fact that disparities and inequities exist in healthcare, but these studies confirmed my worries for cancer patients seeking proton radiation. Although these studies were evaluated from publications within the United States, access to proton treatment is also a barrier in other countries, as it was for the Melling family.

For example, there isn't an operating proton center in Canada.

So, when Derek Tsang, MD, Radiation Oncologist at the Princess Margaret Cancer Centre in Toronto, Canada, prescribes proton radiation for a patient, his only option is to send his patients to one of five proton treatment centers in the United States that the province of Ontario approved for treatments. These centers are in Boston, Massachusetts, Cincinnati, Ohio, Chicago, Illinois, Philadelphia, Pennsylvania, and Jacksonville, Florida. Dr. Tsang's patients and families need to travel thousands of miles for treatment, not to mention obtain time off from work, arrange overnight stays, meals, and more, which adds to the complexity of the prescribed treatments and the potential for socioeconomic disparities.

Because of this geographic challenge, Dr. Tsang and his patients have a lot to consider when deciding on the use of proton treatments. Dr. Tsang is upfront with his patients and families about treatment options. To address the questions of some patients who've inquired about protons, Dr. Tsang explains to patients the rate of tumor control is the same between the two modalities: photon and proton.

As Dr. Tsang mentioned, a patient can truly benefit from proton treatments with the reduction in late-stage toxicities "which is paramount in kids and highly functional adults." When Dr. Tsang recommends proton treatment, he and his patients have a difficult decision to make. As part of the referral process, it's hard to know if a patient can afford the treatments. Proton treatments in the United States cost Canadian patients $225,000 per patient. Although this cost is covered by public health insurance, the incidental, non-medical costs of travel can add up. Access is a challenge not only for the patient and family, but also an added concern for the physician on the patient's behalf.

In contrast, Japan, a country the size of Montana, has eleven proton centers. Clinical trials for proton radiation started in 1979 at the National Institute of Radiological Science. By the year 2000, proton radiation was no longer considered experimental for cancer treatment. Prostate and liver cancer was the most treated disease types. What is interesting is that proton beam therapy is the preferred treatment for head, neck, and pediatric cancers in Japan.

According to the article, "Proton Beam Therapy: Current and Future Status," by Sakurai, Hideyuki:

"Complex structures such as the eyes, optic nerves and central nervous system are close to the base of the skull and the nasal and paranasal cavities. As PBT (proton beam therapy) can reduce the radiation dose to these critical structures, PBT has been traditionally used more than X-ray beam (photon) RT for these cancers... Long-term adverse effects seriously affect the quality of life of pediatric patients. Results from studies promote the use of PBT in pediatric patients."

In Phoebe Melling's case, at first, she was going to be treated with photon therapy, but this would have exposed her whole brain and spinal cord to radiation according to Phoebe's mom, who's also a nurse and spoke through the UMMC video series. As stated, in Japan this is the reason proton is the preferred radiation modality for many pediatric patients. Phoebe's oncologist in Melborne told her mom there were other options. So, her mom began researching and found out there were pediatric patients being treated at MPTC.

Like many proton centers, MPTC offers a concierge service to help patients who travel to receive treatment. MPTC helped the Mellings with lodging, baby seats, cell phones, and even groceries according to the video series. They also offered advice on what do to in the city of Baltimore during their free time.

One of the most thoughtful touches the MPTC team creates for their pediatric patients is they get to choose which type of superhero they want to be and are given a cape to wear during treatments. In addition to the patients' ringing the Hope Bell at the conclusion of their treatments, every pediatric patient is given three wishes at the Magic Castle Princess Land, located in the lobby of the center. The castle was donated by the Children's Cancer Foundation, Inc. Phoebe got to make her three wishes and even celebrate her birthday with the staff at the center. MPTC is truly a magical place to be treated.

At UF Health Proton Therapy Institute in Jacksonville, Florida, pediatric patients also benefit from unique programming such as an education app called Proton U. This is an interactive storybook designed to help prepare patients and families for proton treatments.

Northwestern Medicine Proton Center's child life specialists work with each pediatric patient to help them understand proton therapy and what to expect. They even have a toy the patients could use to push the doll through the CT scan used during treatments.

If I had three wishes that could come true, I'd wish all of them would somehow fix our healthcare system so disparities and inequities in patient care could be eliminated and all people could have access to proton treatment. Between the government-run Canadian healthcare system and our free-market healthcare system, there needs to be a better road to treatment for patients. Yet, once a patient finds protons, the next step is paying for it.

INSURANCE COVERAGE

———

"In our experience, around 85 percent of patients are approved for coverage by their insurance provider. Some private insurance companies cover proton therapy for specific disease sites (cancer types) or on a case-by-case basis."

—MARYLAND PROTON TREATMENT CENTER

Patients I've met through my advocacy work and others have commented on social media that they didn't ask their doctor about proton radiation, as they assumed their insurance wouldn't cover it—but this isn't always the case.

After a patient receives a prescription for proton radiation, the patient's physician will submit a request to the patient's insurance provider to pay for the services prescribed. This process is called **prior authorization** (PA), also sometimes called a pre-authorization.

According to the American Medical Association (AMA), the prior authorization process is the insurance company's **"cost-control process"** in which doctors must request and obtain approval from a health plan before the specific service, treatment, or test is provided to the patient. And it's seemingly a big challenge for doctors and patients alike. I know all about it. I went through the process, and it wore me out.

After my diagnosis and mastectomy, the prior authorization process was the most stressful part of having cancer. Like many patients, I didn't know anything about this process until I was in the thick of it.

In March of 2020, American Society of Clinical Oncology (ASCO) Chair of the Board Monica M. Bertagnolli, MD, FACS, FASCO, spoke about the cost of prior authorization to patients and providers.

"From the time of notification of a required prior authorization through to an ultimate decision being rendered, precious hours and days—sometimes weeks—are slipping away from a patient whose disease may be progressing, whose symptoms may be spiraling out of control, and who may be losing hope for a cure."

How often are insurance authorizations causing a delay in starting radiation treatments?

In a 2019 American Society for Radiation Oncology (ASTRO) survey, nine in ten radiation oncologists report treatment delays due to the insurance process:

"Both academic and private practice radiation oncologists named prior authorization **as the greatest challenge facing the field.**"

In 2017, gynecologic-oncologist, Dr. Boulay titled his blog on KevinMD.com, *"Dear Insurance Doctor: You are not my peer."* In his blog he wrote about his experiences as a physician in cancer care. He said:

"At least weekly, and occasionally daily, insurance companies deny payment for some cancer treatments I prescribe."

He explained he can't recall a time in his career when something in the cancer care continuum hadn't been denied: surgery, chemotherapy, CT, PET scans, and more. Dr. Boulay posits questions like: How can a doctor within an insurance company with no specialty training in oncology be the person authorized to approve or deny cancer treatments he was prescribing for his patients?

From my research and physician interviews, it's frustrating for doctors and patients alike to wait for the peer at the insurance company to review the medical case, especially when the peer really isn't a peer in the medical specialty of the doctor prescribing treatment!

This problem isn't just in cancer care.

In an article titled *"Inside Cleveland Clinics $10M Prior-Authorization Price Tag,"* Andis Robeznieks reported that in 2018 the Cleveland Clinic expected to process nine hundred thousand outpatient prior authorization requests, which takes time away from caring for patients. Between hold time on the phone to unanswered faxes, some faxes sent six times per patient, the downstream costs add up. In 2018 the Cleveland Clinic projected it to add up to $10 million up from $9.7 million in 2017 and $9 million in 2015.

What a lot of time spent chasing the insurance companies for answers.

It's clear from this survey and my own experience, even with my insurance company representative never meeting me or examining me, that my insurance company was and still is part of my medical care team through the prior authorization process.

Insurance providers make decisions on whether to pay for treatments and tests according to their policies. But, as I soon found out, sometimes their decisions can be challenged.

When I received my prescription for protons, the cost of being treated with protons and photons was the same so I was hopeful my treatments would be approved. Yet, one of the very first questions I asked Dr. Eblan:

"Will insurance pay for my treatment?"

Dr. Eblan explained he would submit my case for prior authorization, but I might not be approved on the first try.

To illustrate this, the New York Proton Center's website is a great resource for patients seeking answers about insurance coverage. According to their site, each patient's coverage is determined by their insurance policy, clinical history, medical diagnosis, and other factors such as how many treatments will be required.

As for patients with Medicare coverage, I found through research on Medicare.gov that in general, proton radiation treatment is covered by Medicare, Medicaid, *and* some private insurance companies.

Sometimes this process takes a few steps before insurance will pay for the proton treatments or not. However, these steps can happen in days, weeks, or even many months at a time.

You'll see this play out through the patient stories later in this book where many of us ended up getting our treatments approved and covered by our insurance providers, yet our cancer care was delayed! For example, in the three stories about breast cancer, all our cases got approved. It took a while, in weeks and months, but our doctors advocated for us, and our insurance providers overturned our cases.

PRIOR AUTHORIZATION PROCESS

The prior authorization process can be extremely frustrating (to put it lightly) for physicians and patients as described earlier in the ASTRO data. However, if prescribed proton treatment, the cancer center teams and physicians understand the process and will advocate for a patient's treatment plan to be approved.

Outlined below are potential steps in the insurance approval process.

PRIOR AUTHORIZATION SUBMISSION AND DENIAL—1ST APPEAL

If the physician's first submission for approval is denied by the insurance provider, the physician may appeal the case.

Sometimes, doctors will submit a "letter of medical necessity" (LMN) or a "comparative case" on the patient's behalf. In each scenario, the doctor may provide additional information supporting the recommendation for proton radiation treatment. During this process, I recommend keeping track of all the correspondences from the insurance company and the cancer center.

According to the nonprofit Kaiser Family Foundation article by Tom Murphy which analyzed data on care sought inside an insurer's coverage network, health insurers denied nearly forty-three million claims in 2017 in the individual insurance market and only **1 percent of patients appealed** those decisions. The study further stated that patients gave up because they said they were "intimidated by the process or don't have the energy" because of their treatment. That's so sad, yet many of the patients I interviewed for this book, appealed their cases and many of our cases were overturned and insurance paid for our treatments!

WAITING TO HEAR BACK FROM 1ST APPEAL

When I was treated with protons, I was on my husband's insurance plan but didn't know what type of policy his company had with the insurance company. Our contact at the Maryland Proton Treatment Center (MPTC) told us to talk to the Human Resources (HR) Manager at my husband's company to find out what type of policy we had. Getting the HR person involved at the beginning can save precious time when attempting to get treatments approved.

If the employer has a self-funded, or self-insured plan, it means the employer assumes the financial risk for providing health care benefits to its employees. Self-insured employers pay for claims out-of-pocket as they are presented instead of paying a predetermined premium to an insurance provider for a fully insured plan.

According to HCAA's *Self-Funding Primer*, if a patient's insurance coverage is through a self-funded plan, the employer has the option to cover the cost of the treatment for the patient. Later in this book, you'll see firsthand when two patients' proton treatments were denied, two employers decided to pay for their treatments!

PEER TO PEER REVIEW PROCESS

As Dr. Boulay said in his blog when he was attempting to get a PET scan approved for his patient by the **peer** at the insurance provider, he asked if the doctor was a gynecologic oncologist. The doctor said no, they practiced family medicine. Dr. Boulay explained that a previous PET scan had caught two lesions that were not seen on the CT scan. Despite

Dr. Boulay's request for the PET, the **peer** approved a CT and declined to cover the PET scan for the patient.

Dr. Boulay closed his blog on the peer-to-peer review process with the following questions:

"Didn't we have the same idealistic view of changing the world one patient at a time? Didn't we take the same oath that began 'primum non nocere'—first do no harm? So, when did our paths diverge?"

I thought the same thing when I spoke to Allison and Dr. Eblan, when they told me a radiation oncologist was not first reviewing my case.

After my initial decline for coverage, Dr. Eblan appealed and requested a **peer-to-peer review** of my case. This meant he was speaking to a doctor at the insurance company to review my case to approve coverage or not. Except in my case, and in many, the doctor who first reviewed my case at United-Healthcare wasn't a **radiation oncologist.**

While this was happening, my stress increased. Many patients like me asked: Should I keep fighting insurance with my doctor's support?

Based on my experience with my own insurance denials and appeals, I don't use the word "fighting" lightly.

On May 2, 2018, I received a letter from UnitedHealthcare, they had reviewed the appeal regarding coverage of the services to receive from the MPTC and stated they knew I wanted the decision reconsidered.

Further along in the same letter, UnitedHealthcare provided details on what they considered a life-threatening sickness or condition. As I read the letter in angered me.

"Please note if you have a life-threatening sickness or condition (one that is likely to cause death within one year of the request for treatment), UnitedHealthcare with your employer may at its discretion, consider an otherwise unproven service to be a Covered Health Service for that sickness or condition."

They closed the letter abruptly.

"Our prior payment decision for this service is therefore unchanged. You are responsible for all costs related to this service(s)."

Just like that, UnitedHealthcare denied coverage for my treatments.

This is exactly when my pain became my purpose to help others.

With Dr. Eblan's help, we kept going.

APPEAL AND WAIT AGAIN

Dr. Eblan called me and together we decided to appeal a third and final time. For this appeal, Dr. Eblan submitted a nine-page letter of medical necessity and a comparative case study as to why proton treatment was more beneficial than photon (IMRT) for my case. He outlined in detail my clinical history, my family's clinical history, facts about the impact on the heart, ribs, and lungs using photon (IMRT) radiation exiting the body versus proton being more targeted. The opening line in Dr. Eblan's letter to UnitedHealthcare:

"I am requesting an **expedited appeal process**. Ms. Durgin can't wait weeks for an answer to start treatments given her surgery was two months ago on March 6, 2018. Additionally, I am requesting a **radiation oncologist** evaluate this request for proton beam therapy for Ms. Durgin's treatment of breast cancer."

In the meantime, Dr. Eblan and my oncologist wanted my proton treatments to start four weeks, no more than six weeks after surgery. It had already been eight weeks. Further, according to breastcancer.org, if chemotherapy isn't part of the treatment plan as it wasn't for me, external beam radiation, like protons, should begin about "three to six weeks after surgery."

I felt time was running out.

I called Dr. Eblan on Friday, May 4, 2018 and told him I would pay out of pocket for protons. He decided to schedule my first treatment on the following Monday, May 7, 2018. I told Dr. Eblan that I planned on fighting my way through this process with UnitedHealthcare until they would approve payment.

I wasn't going away. I spent many years in sales and marketing at Marriott International, and as a result I knew a lot of people in the media. I considered telling them my story and asking for their help. My friend Joanne Haight suggested we march to UnitedHealthcare headquarters in pink t-shirts, demanding to be heard. I was so angry and not just for me but for all the people I imagined this happening to in the United States. Meanwhile, my cancer was potentially spreading—that's why I needed treatment to begin with!

Later that same day on May 4, 2018, Dr. Eblan called me and said, "Ms. Durgin, your treatment is approved by United-Healthcare." I cried. I wanted to give Dr. Eblan and Allison Scull a hug of gratitude. I would never be able to explain how grateful I felt for their tireless work on my behalf. They are amazing and they continue help patients through this process of denials and appeals even as I publish this book.

Yet as happy as I was, I was also angry that the prior authorization and appeals process created such a significant bottleneck and delay in my treatment plan. I knew I needed to do more to help educate and inform others of this frustrating and seemingly broken process. I wanted to provide hope that many times are cases are overturned and the story has a positive ending.

A week after I **started** treatment, my insurance story ended, at least for protons, as I received a letter from UnitedHealthcare:

"We sent you a letter on May 2, 2018. **This is a correction to that letter**. We've reviewed the appeal again and made changes because we completed our **specialty review**, and our previous decision has changed."

Why couldn't they have done a specialty review in the first place?

Where is the accountability for insurance providers in this process?

Abruptly the decision was overturned, and my insurance approved twenty-eight days of proton treatments! If you think this sounds exhausting, it is. But not just for the patient, for the physician and patient support team as well.

In 2019, according to a survey by ASTRO of seven hundred radiation oncologists, 93 percent of patients are delayed from lifesaving treatments due to the peer-to-peer review within the prior authorization process.

Mark V. Mishra, MD, Radiation Oncologist, Associate Professor of Radiation Oncology and Director of Radiation Oncology Clinical Research, University of Maryland School of Medicine mentioned the prior authorization challenges when I interviewed him:

"It's discouraging and disappointing that some patients don't have access and they're blocked from getting proton beam therapy or blocked from even participating in a clinical trial."

Yet I remain hopeful as more cancer centers open that the insurance prior authorization process will improve and patients can more easily access protons for their cancer care.

HOW DOES THE PROTON
MACHINE WORK?

———

"Imagine a world without fear of cancer. We do."

—VARIAN

Varian is one of five manufacturers of the proton beam system. According to their website, in 1948 with just six employees and $22,000 of capital, Varian Associates was founded by a group of scientists with connections to Stanford University. Over the years the company innovated, acquired various companies, and expanded its product offerings in radiotherapy and other related technologies. In 2007, Varian entered the proton beam market when it acquired ACCEL systems, a privately held manufacturer of proton therapy systems. In the same year, Varian entered the Fortune list of one thousand top companies.

Through my advocacy work with the Alliance for Proton Therapy Access, I met a few of the people who work for Varian Proton Solutions at Varian Medical Systems. From talking to them and learning more about Varian, I know their commitment to fight cancer is real. It's not just a statement for marketing purposes. The company is equally passionate about their people, products, customers, and the community.

As part of their community commitment and the commitment to their employees, I shared my story with breast cancer and how I found the Varian ProBeam machine at the Maryland Proton Treatment Center (MPTC). I thanked the team for their hard work and ingenuity through a Zoom meeting during the COVID-19 pandemic. The Varian team played a significant role in saving my life! Sharing my story meant so much to me. I'm forever grateful for their technology.

Almost three years out of treatment and through publishing this book, I learned a lot more about my own treatment at MPTC. I reached out to Varian as I wanted to know more about the ProBeam machine. I interviewed Deepak "Dee" Khuntia, MD, Senior Vice President, Chief Medical Officer at Varian.

I asked Dr. Khuntia a few questions I thought might be helpful for patients to know. Starting with:

How does the Varian machine compare with other proton machines?

"One of the major differentiating features of Varian technology is that we use a technology called intensity modulated proton therapy (IMPT) that allows us to rapidly 'paint' the radiation dose with a very fine brush…almost pixelating the tumor volume. This allows us to have a more conformal radiation treatment plan which means it shapes the radiation beams to closely fit the area of the cancer. The Varian ProBeam system also has one of the most powerful cyclotrons on the market which allows the system to deliver radiation in a very short time. Given our world class expertise in imaging and treatment plans, we have been able to bring state-of-the-art image guidance with cone beam CT imaging and treatment planning. That is extremely specific to our machines, which allows for high precision and higher quality treatment deliveries."

Dr. Khuntia helped me understand more about the machine used at the proton center when I asked:

What type of machine was used during my cancer treatment at Maryland Proton Treatment Center?

"The Maryland system is a five-room ProBeam system with the most advanced form of pencil beam scanning used for IMPT treatments. The system is powered by a superconducting cyclotron which accelerates protons to 60 percent the speed of light. Superconductivity is used in MRI machines as well to create very powerful magnetic fields at low power consumption. In proton therapy, the magnetic field is not used for imaging, and does not reach the patient, but to bend the protons on a circular track for acceleration, hence the name 'cyclotron.' Protons are being generated from water, first to hydrogen gas, and then later in the process ionized to single protons. A single glass of water contains enough protons to treat all cancer patients for the foreseeable future! Protons are then transported in a vacuum tube to the treatment room, where a scanning system is used to aim the 'pencil beam' with sub-millimeter precision to the tumor."

This technology is simply amazing to me. I don't think I can ever look at a glass of water the same way!

During the treatment planning phase, I had the chance to tour MPTC and see the cyclotron, the heart of the ProBeam. I decided not to visit the machine. It was too intimidating to me. Now I know why! Learning the cyclotron weighs ninety tons, almost the weight of an airplane, is intimidating.

Dr. Khuntia described the treatment planning phase which is one of the first appointments patients go through prior to treatments at a proton center.

"One of the most important aspects of the process is the treatment planning phase. Based on high resolution 3D images of the tumor and surrounding healthy tissues, an incredibly detailed plan is created. That results in a set of 'instructions' for the delivery system. The treatment planning system (TPS)—in this case called Varian Eclipse TPS—optimizes the delivery plan to make it as precise (conformal) as possible, while at the same time being quick to deliver."

So that explains why on most days my treatments were roughly twenty minutes, and some days were longer if the center was busy, and the machine was needed to treat a pediatric patient.

Given the complexity and sophistication of the machine, I was curious to hear:

How long does it take to build a proton machine?

"It takes roughly a year to build the ProBeam equipment in the factory, and in parallel the infrastructure is developed on the site where the ProBeam will be housed. After that the system is shipped, installed, and commissioned by Varian. That takes another eight to twelve months based on the configuration of the system (single-room versus multi-room)."

From the initial purchase of the machine to delivery, it takes roughly three hundred people from all different roles at Varian including purchasing, manufacturing, installation, service, and training. According to Dr. Khuntia, to produce a proton machine, it costs roughly ten times as much as a photon machine.

Because of the weight of the machine's parts, transporting the parts by air isn't feasible, so Varian ships the ProBeam equipment by road and boat in heavy shipping containers.

By the time the proton machine is available to a patient for treatment, it can cost an estimated **two times the amount of money than photon treatments.** So, the more patients are treated with protons, the investment in the system pays off. But if insurance companies keep declining authorizations for treatments, demand for protons could decrease. This seems so unjust.

Dr. Khuntia explained the proton therapy systems have a lifetime of twenty years or longer and are decommissioned after that period.

According to Minesh Mehta, MD, in *Imaging and Technology News,* Varian set its sights on the future of proton therapy by developing the ProBeam 360 which uses the same precision but is smaller in size so it can make proton therapy more accessible and more affordable.

I'm so grateful for Varian and their commitment to a "world without fear of cancer." It makes me shiver to say those words out loud.

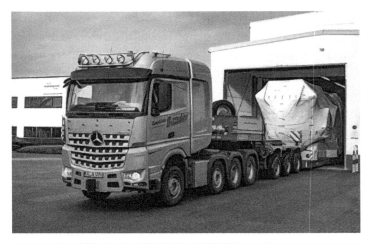

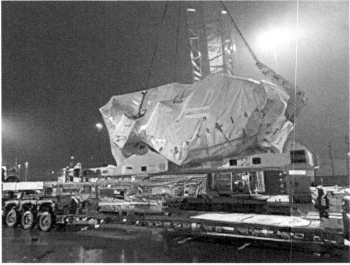

Picture of the ProBeam machine en route, courtesy of Varian.

COST SAVINGS, HIGHER QUALITY OF CARE? THE RADIATION ONCOLOGY (RO) ALTERNATIVE PAYMENT MODEL (APM)

"The National Cancer Institute estimates the costs of cancer therapy in 2010 in the United States reached more than $124 billion, representing 5 percent of total health care spending; the figure is projected to reach $157 billion by 2020. In 2010, the most expensive cancers to treat were breast ($16.5 billion), colorectal ($14.1 billion), lymphoma ($12.1 billion), lung ($12.1 billion), and prostate ($11.9 billion)."

These facts and figures are eye opening and are found in the forty-two-page report, "United States Department of Health and Human Services Report to Congress: Episodic Alternative Payment Model for Radiation Therapy Services" from November 2017.

Since 2014, with the cost of cancer rising, the Center for Medicaid and Medicare Services (CMS), which is part of the Department of Health and Human Services in the United States, has sought ways to reduce the cost of cancer care.

According to Medicare.gov, in the United States, Medicare provides health insurance for people sixty-five and older and people under sixty-five with certain disabilities. Depending on the type of Medicare policy a person buys, it provides coverage for things like, basic health services, including hospital stays, physician services, prescription drugs, and cancer treatments like radiation therapy (RT) services. It works similarly to private insurance in that a deductible must be met before Medicare will pay for medical expenses.

According to the CMS.gov newsroom, currently, if a patient with Medicare is prescribed proton radiation and is approved for treatment, the patient would be billed for each service rendered. This is what is known as fee for service payment. The Radiation Oncology Alternative Payment Model (RO-APM) would seek to change the way the physician bills for services. Instead of a fee for service, CMS proposed to test an episode-based payment model. In layman's terms, this means a fixed price or bundled price for all the services rendered during an episode of radiation treatment.

An episode starts from the initial consultation. It then moves to the radiation mapping appointment which can last up to an hour where the physician and radiation team determine where the radiation dose would be distributed for each patient. Then treatments begin. Depending on the diagnosis, a patient can be prescribed daily treatments, sometimes twice a day, that can be as short as a couple of weeks in time to over a month of treatments. When treatment concludes, the patient visits the doctor to see how the patient is progressing. As part of this process some patients get scans to see if the cancer was eradicated.

Under the proposed RO-APM, this entire process would be associated with a fixed price for treatment over a ninety-day period. So, in my case, my first consultation with Dr. Eblan was in March of 2018. By the time I finished treatments and went to see Dr. Eblan for my fist follow up appointment, over ninety days had passed, most of which was waiting for my insurance provider to approve my case.

Officially, on December 28, 2015, Congress passed the Patient Access and Medicare Protection Act (PAMPA), which required the Secretary of Health and Human Services to submit to Congress a report on "the development of an episodic alternative payment model" (APM) for RT services. The final Report to Congress is forty-two pages and was published in November 2017—the same report cited at the start of this chapter.

In a nutshell, the goal of the new payment model would test whether a national base rate versus a fee for service would reduce Medicare spending while preserving or improving the quality of care for Medicare patients. The RO-APM model focuses on quality of care and links payments to reporting and performance on quality measures, clinical data reporting, and patient experience as factors when determining payment to RO-APM participants.

According to CMS.gov, the RO-APM is projected to save CMS $320 million over the next five years. IMRT and proton beam therapy are included in the new payment model as are other radiation modalities. There are sixteen cancer types included: anal, breast, head and neck, pancreatic, bladder, cervical, liver, prostate, lung, upper GI, colorectal, and uterine cancers, lymphoma, CNS tumors, bone metastases, and brain metastases.

CMS invited professional societies and those interested to provide comments and recommendations to the proposed ruling.

The American Hospital Association (AHA) and the American Society for Radiation Oncology (ASTRO) weighed in on the recommended test model. On September 19, 2019, the AHA submitted a nineteen-page letter to Ms. Seema Verna who at the time was the head of CMS. The AHA represents five thousand member hospitals, health systems, and other health care organizations, clinician partners—including more than 270,000 affiliated physicians, two million nurses and other caregivers—and the 43,000 health care leaders who belong with their professional memberships. In summary, AHA supports a more innovative approach to more "accountable and streamlined care." However, the AHA believed there were many flaws in the proposed new RO-APM test. Concerns included a potential reduction in patient access for radiation therapy and a national base price for re-imbursement the AHA was seeking more transparency to understand how the pricing process was derived.

On the same day, ASTRO submitted a forty-one-page letter to Ms. Seema Verna from which 1.4 million healthcare providers and others were involved. ASTRO stated their support of some elements of the RO-APM test and like the AHA, disagreed with other proponents of the test namely, CMS's payment cuts of $320 million over five years.

ASTRO stated the RO-APM:

> "Would jeopardize **access** to safe and effective radiation treatments by putting too much financial strain on radiation oncology practices that have no choice but to participate. Of great concern is the impact that this will have on access to needed health care services, especially for beneficiaries in rural and underserved areas. Because, in the end, if these detrimental cuts are implemented, those who suffer the most will be patients."

In 2019, I heard about the RO-APM through my work as a volunteer proton advocate at the Alliance for Proton Therapy Access. I was concerned the new ruling would reduce access to proton therapy. How much more difficult can it be for cancer patients seeking this treatment? As proton volunteers and patients, we discussed our concerns and the Alliance's involvement toward this ruling.

On September 16, 2019, the Alliance also submitted a letter to Ms. Seema Verna expressing concerns for the new payment model specifically for proton radiation. The new national base case proposed by CMS would put cancer patients at risk as it would not come close to covering the cost of proton radiation for Medicare patients. It also stated that the data used for the report submitted to Congress included outdated data on the efficacy of proton beam therapy.

Again, Medicare is the federal health insurance program for people sixty-five and older in the United States. There are different plans people can choose from. In general, proton radiation has been covered under various Medicare plans depending on the cancer diagnosis and whether the treatments are inpatient or outpatient. When I talked to patients who had insurance coverage under Medicare, their proton radiation treatments were approved on the first submission. Changing to the RO-APM could be devastating to some of these patients.

On September 18, 2020, CMS released their final ruling on the RO-APM and adopted changes, concluding that they seem minor and not enough to prevent a potential devastating impact to patients. The five-year test would begin on July 1, 2021, instead of January 1, 2021.

Tyler Blackwell, MD, Medical Physicist at Radformation has clinical experience in radiation therapy. Dr. Blackwell wrote about the changes on the Radformation website, "The new payment structure may ultimately reshape how departments care for patients. With a nationwide implementation, the effects will be broad, but could result in disparate effects depending on geography and patient makeup."

When I interviewed Dr. Bajaj in December of 2020, he was also concerned about the RO-APM:

"For some facilities that are in the process of considering proton therapy as a service line for patients, the RO-APM will serve as a death knell to innovation in radiation oncology. Ironically, it's the *innovation arm* of CMS (CMMI) that is essentially thwarting the adoption and capital investment in technologies which will move the field forward and have the potential greatest impact on survivorship. All the new technologies and treatment modalities in our specialty come with a requirement for more capital, overhead, and staffing resources. At some point the calculus of reimbursement cuts from federal sources, if appreciably Draconian, will slow the pace of both adoption and further innovation. There is already a limited number of these types of innovations available in the landscape now, so the issues of equity and access to advanced treatment modalities will only be further magnified."

On March 1, 2021, the Community of Oncology Alliance, which is made up of radiation oncologists, members of the radiation oncology cancer care team, group practices, hospitals, patient advocates, device manufacturers, and others authored a letter to the Biden administration regarding concerns over the RO-APM. They shared similar concerns as mentioned, specifically the new model is too focused on achieving significant savings, at the risk of hurting access to care and quality.

The RO-APM was initiated under the Obama administration. The proposed work continued through the Trump administration and thereafter. On the eleventh anniversary of the Affordable Care Act, on March 23, 2021, President Biden toured a proton therapy center. The transcript of his interview at the site is posted on the Whitehouse.gov website. President Biden stated protecting healthy tissues is one of the main reasons to focus on proton radiation.

Many of us who advocate for patient access to protons were hopeful after hearing President Biden speak. Yet so far, his administration hasn't made any changes to the start test date of July 1, 2021. We were hopeful the President would weigh in and consider the recommendations from societies that took the time to respond to the proposed changes.

But, a glimmer of hope is on the horizon! On May 25, 2021, the Senate confirmed Chiquita Brooks-LaSure as the next CMS administrator. During her confirmation testimony on April 15 2021, she stated:

> *"If confirmed, I will work to make the programs overseen by CMS work better together to help the people they serve. Medicare, Medicaid, and coverage on the Marketplaces remain the pillars of our health care system, and there is much we can do to strengthen those programs to improve quality, lower costs, and expand access."*

I couldn't be any more hopeful after hearing these words. July 1, 2021 is right around the corner. I can't wait to see her commitment play out for patients seeking radiation care, including proton therapy. We'll be watching.

CLINICAL TRIALS

———

I'm one of the 8 percent!

At my first consultation with Dr. Eblan, he told me about two clinical trials investigating proton radiation benefits in breast cancer. I enrolled in both without hesitation because I felt so grateful for people before me who enrolled in clinical trials. Without their participation, I might not have had the chance to be treated with protons. Because of this, I knew right away no matter what it took, I wanted to pay it forward for other breast cancer patients who would benefit from my data included in the studies.

I also thought about women before me who enrolled in clinical trials for the drug Tamoxifen, which many breast cancer patients like me take to prevent recurrence of cancer. I'm so thankful for those women, too. I don't even know them, but because of their courage, I enrolled in the proton trials and later in another trial with Tamoxifen and the drug Ibrance.

Yet, I didn't know at the time only 8 percent of all cancer patients enroll in trials.

From a patient's viewpoint, I can understand why people don't enroll in trials as there are many factors which influence a patient's decision. Imperial Clinical Resources made a list of twenty-five, and I've summarized some of the key points below and included my own feedback:

- Lack of awareness.
- Insurance doesn't approve proton radiation treatments, so the patient can't enroll in the trial, which is incredibly challenging and unjust if you ask me.
- Cost of travel and potential overnight stays during the clinical trial.
- Lack of understanding.
- Risk of side effects.
- Patient doesn't qualify for the trial.
- Physician is unaware of the trial and/or is not interested in participating.
- Can't get time off from work for additional clinical trial appointments.
- Uncomfortable with what's being asked of the patient. In my case, the clinical trial director and my doctor had to take pictures of my breast and the skin in the treated area.
- Unsupportive family, friends, or care team.
- Might get the placebo, or may be in the control arm and not receive the potential lifesaving drug for the trial.

As a patient, I enrolled in three clinical trial trials. I learned about the trials as I was being treated.

According to the Food and Drug Administration here (FDA), it typically takes an average of three to seven years for a medical device to be approved by the FDA, compared with an average of twelve years for drugs.

In the article "The Evolution of Proton Therapy: Accelerating Cancer Treatment" on Proton Therapy Technologies website, a superconducting cyclotron—in layman's terms, a proton radiation machine—is a good example of a medical device born through the exploration of particles and nuclear physics in the 1930s, researched in the 1940s, tested on patients in the 1950s, and then approved by the FDA for cancer treatments since 1988.

According to the National Comprehensive Cancer Network, clinical trials are done when there is "good reason to believe a new test or treatment may improve the care of patients."

Clinical trials have different phases beginning at phase zero which, according to the American Cancer Society, "may help researchers find out if the drugs do what they're expected to do" and therefore can move to the next phases which are phases one through three. After phase two or three, a drug, for example, can be submitted to the (FDA) if it has met all the phase requirements for the FDA submission. Phase four studies evaluate studies over a longer period of time. For example, one of the clinical trials I'm enrolled in is a ten-year trial.

Knowing which phase their trial is in is important for patients. The higher the phase, the more is known about the study. Patients can visit clinicaltrials.gov and find trials that are recruiting, in progress, and completed.

In my physician interviews, I was curious to know more about clinical trials and protons.

What are the challenges?

Mark V. Mishra, MD, Radiation Oncologist, Associate Professor of Radiation Oncology and Director of Radiation Oncology Clinical Research, University of Maryland School of Medicine shared his sentiments:

"It's challenging as we have barriers within the insurance company and not just for the treatment, but also with clinical trials *and* proton treatment. This impedes progress in that way. "

Deepak "Dee" Khuntia, MD, Senior Vice President, Chief Medical Officer at Varian explained the progress that's been made just in the last year:

"We have seen data showing patients with proton therapy have a lower incidence of secondary cancers, advanced tumors receiving chemotherapy with proton therapy have lower side effects versus standard radiation, and we have seen improved outcomes with tumors such as liver tumors." This is great news!

I also asked J. Isabelle Choi, MD, Radiation Oncologist, Clinical Director, and Director of Research at the New York Proton Center and Carl Rossi, MD, Radiation Oncologist, Medical Director at California Proton Therapy Center the following question:

What should a patient know about clinical trials?

Dr. Choi responded:

"Proton therapy is a more costly treatment compared with traditional radiation therapy due to the more intricate machinery and technology required to deliver the proton particle accurately and precisely. The **proton** particle is larger and charged, in comparison with the much smaller, noncharged **photon** particle used to deliver traditional radiation therapy. Due to this initial cost disparity between the two modalities, it has become much more challenging to provide patients who would benefit from this technology with access to proton therapy due to barriers in insurance coverage for proton therapy."

Dr. Choi also mentioned the cost of managing side effects or possible cancer recurrence is not factored into the decision to treat the patient with proton therapy, and said, "These (side effects) are likely substantially less with proton therapy due to the decrease in normal tissue exposure with protons compared with photons."

Dr. Choi continued:

"We have data already that shows where dose is being distributed, and that it is much less to non-target tissue with protons compared with photons, which then lends itself to the basic understanding that toxicity will be spared to these tissues. This is what we have always attempted to achieve in radiation oncology—to spare unnecessary radiation dose and therefore toxicities to normal tissues. However, because we need to justify the increased cost of proton therapy to allow our patients access to this **superior technology**, we have invested many resources into developing these clinical trials. It will also be important to obtain this data to best allocate our proton resources to those patients who will benefit the most.

"Insurance providers can have different rules and regulations within and between different states, and across insurance providers, there are very disparate authorization policies. Therefore, it is difficult to say patients will always have a better likelihood of insurance approval if they are on a clinical trial, but, depending on the specific insurance provider, there is a possibility there may be an exception made for patients participating on a clinical trial to not impede the furthering of medical knowledge through research."

Dr. Rossi responded:

"In the case of proton therapy, I'm not a big fan of requiring prospective randomized trials as the only 'level of evidence' before adapting a new treatment or technology, saying we've got to do prospective randomized trials before you can do XYZ. The reason, if you look at how radiation therapy has developed, [it's] not the same as saying we're testing a new drug that we need to test against an existing drug with a different mechanism of action. We've done all our advances in radiation therapy over the last one hundred plus years based on physics, and this is just another step along those same roads. So, if you're going to go into a clinical trial, and you're potentially being randomized between X-rays and protons, and you're getting the same total radiation dose to the cancer, I have a little problem with that, because what you're doing is you're just randomizing people to receiving more or less of a known toxin to see if there's a clinical difference, in effect. Can you get away with it? Despite the fact we've known for over a century, **radiation is a toxin and the less you receive the better**. Would you enroll in such a trial? We certainly do trials to try to optimize our therapy, how much to give for a particular diagnosis and in how many fractions, but I vehemently disagree with the idea you have to do a randomized trial between X-rays and protons before you can use protons in a clinical context."

That said, results from recent completed trials are exciting! In 2019 at the American Society for Radiation Oncology (ASTRO) annual conference, Brian C. Baumann, MD, of Washington University School of Medicine discussed a significant finding with protons.

Dr. Baumann, summarized the findings in a comparative effectiveness analysis at the University of Pennsylvania and determined that this study shows the "potential to escalate the intensity of chemo radiotherapy and that in turn may improve outcomes."

In the years ahead, the escalation in layman's terms means the potential to increase the dose of radiation, or dose up the protons due to less side effects. The dose up effect may in fact increase a patient's survival versus photons. More studies are needed, but this was exciting for me to learn!

I asked Arpit Chhabra, MD, Radiation Oncologist and Director of Education at the New York Proton Center, if I understood it correctly. If the side effects are better with protons and the survival rate is the same, could physicians increase the dose of proton radiation to be able to affect the survival rate?

Dr. Chhabra explained:

"When delivering equivalent radiation doses, the unique property of proton therapy allows the potential for less side effects than photons. Therefore, this presents an opportunity to take the dose higher with protons, because we believe this may enhance survival. This is what certain studies in lung cancer and glioblastoma are currently attempting to study."

It's exciting that patients were willing to be enrolled in the studies we discussed. These studies will lead to potential future studies to show the difference between overall survival with proton radiation versus photon radiation, which would be a significant breakthrough for cancer patients and the field of oncology.

THE PATIENT EXPERIENCE

———

"If you're going to have breast cancer, you got the good kind."

—MY NURSE

My cancer journey in some ways is like other patients I've spoken to. One day we're living our lives and the next day we find out we have cancer. Our world flips in one conversation; suddenly our own mortality is front and center. Some might even say life as we knew it wouldn't be the same. We're suddenly thrown into digesting the diagnosis, finding a new physician team, and booking appointments for tests, all the while wondering if the cancer is spreading.

Within a matter of days or weeks, we are tossed into new relationships with physicians we've just met. We're at our most vulnerable state and, in an instant, we need to trust the new doctors' advice. Physicians are the experts on curing us and healing us. They've dedicated their lives to helping others and have taken an oath of ethics to do no harm. They're inspiring and sometimes intimidating all the same.

Yet as patients in cancer care, we arrive at the doctor's office without training and we're desperate for a cure. We're worried, full of fear, uncertainty, and listen intently for hope things will be okay. This is how the patient and physician relationship begins. Yet, the best doctors know communication and trust are vital to patient healing, clinical outcomes, and the patient experience. To these physicians, compassion and effective communication is just as important as safe, high-quality clinical outcomes. These doctors understand relationships of trust matter.

As John Noseworthy, MD, states in the *New England Journal of Medicine*, "Amid the complexities and changes in health care today, medicine's most fundamental element remains the relationship between patient and physician. This relationship at the heart of health care has been a constant across cultures and centuries, and I believe it must remain central to medical practice even as medicine evolves."

So when I got the call from the nurse that I had cancer and I had the "good kind," I thought, *What the heck is the good kind?*

One thing all of us cancer patients have in common, is how we received the news:

"You have cancer."

I didn't know there was a good kind of cancer. It seemed like an oxymoron. I remember thinking, somehow, I was lucky even though I didn't feel lucky. I think the nurse was trying to lighten the mood and her intentions were good. She explained why she said it was the good kind. I had ductal carcinoma in situ (DCIS). But, hearing the words "you have cancer" is scary. My head was spinning.

I heard the same version of this conversation told in different ways through patients I've met and others written about in this book. There's no doubt medical providers want to soften the blow by using humor or analogies that elicit a silver lining of hope and encouragement.

I can't imagine calling patients day in and day out or seeing them in the office and sharing the heartbreaking and scary news. So, I'm not sure what's right for each patient.

My college roommate Annie was diagnosed with breast cancer in the same exact spot as me four years before my diagnosis. Her recollection of her conversation with her doctor in Boston went something like,

"If you had to get breast cancer, you got the garden variety."

Annie told me she had no idea what it meant, and she's still not sure seven years later.

Eva, a patient I met through the Maryland Proton Treatment Center (MPTC), pulled through roughly seven hours of surgery to remove a tumor on her thymus, she remembered thinking:

"Carcinogen? Isn't that cancerous? Too many tubes were attached to me, and I was too medicated to be thinking about this."

After the initial call and diagnosis, each patient follows a diagnostic process before a plan of care is established and treatment begins. Many times, patients like me moved right into scans—a CT, MRI, or PET scan.

From appointment to appointment, it's an opportunity for a cancer patient (or any patient) to feel comforted, confident, informed, and cared for—or not, depending on the patient and the person serving the patient.

Fast forward from the biopsy in late January of 2018 to May 7, 2018 when I started proton radiation treatment at MPTC. The moment my husband and I arrived MPTC, I knew I was in a place that truly defined patient experience excellence on every level at every customer touch point. I felt so cared for; I even felt special.

At the reception desk, most of us going through treatment got to know Ms. Rose (Roberta). She greeted her patients with hugs. Despite being grown adults, we were her children. Her warm smile and caring ways were like a ray of sunshine each day. If it was raining out or I felt tired, Ms. Rose lifted me up and made me feel like a normal person, not a patient. I can't think about MPTC without thinking about Ms. Rose's beautiful and caring smile.

After checking in and changing into my medical gown, I felt like I moved from business professional to patient, just like that. It was hard to swallow each time I went for treatment.

In the waiting room, I sat with fellow patients waiting for our turn to go to the treatment room. I read my book, chatted with patients, and heard so many patient stories. We were all in the same room together, with our family or friends. It was surreal.

During treatment, radiation therapists are the team who manage the day in and day out of getting patients on and off the radiation table and in position to receive the treatments they deliver. My therapists were amazing! Phillip, Z, Megan, Andrea, and Laruen were efficient and so caring. Each day they smiled with warm compassion as they greeted me in the waiting room and took me to the treatment room. They made me laugh and they played the best music during my treatments. They listened when I told them I felt like a painful lightning bolt of radiation hit my breast on many days. After a while, I didn't say anything as I felt like I was complaining. They would never make anyone feel that way, I was just tired of bringing it up.

After twenty-eight proton treatments, I ended up having three fractured ribs from treatment which were diagnosed by Dr. Eblan about eleven months later. I wonder now if the lightning bolt feeling was the radiation frying my bones. I feel lucky I had protons as maybe this could have been worse with photons. Who knows?

Throughout my appointments with Dr. Eblan, my husband called Dr. Eblan a savant in communication and I agree. Dr Eblan heals through building relationships of trust and compassion. He has the biggest heart and smile. He cares so much. He is gifted in asking questions and digging deep when I needed it and didn't feel like I wanted to speak up. He makes me feel so comfortable and cared for. He's helped me in so many ways just by caring so much. I've sent two patients to Dr. Eblan, and both say the same about his communication style. He defines patient experience excellence on so many levels.

Other patients I spoke with had positive experiences with their radiation oncologists during their initial consults and throughout their treatments. Each provider seemed to build rapport and create relationships which positively affected their experiences and healing.

Frank Rosenthal, a patient I met through the MPTC, was treated for a cancerous tumor at the base of his tongue at the point where it attaches deep in the throat. By the time Frank found out the tumor was cancerous at Stage I, he had been through an attempted robotic surgery to remove the tumor but found out his oral cavity was too small, so he was sent for proton radiation. At MPTC, he was prescribed protons and his doctor told him up front some of the side effects could be brutal. But Frank appreciated his honesty.

Frank had sixty-two proton treatments to treat the lymph nodes in his neck as well as the tumor. Each treatment lasted about fifteen minutes. He had two treatments each day. His experience went well, until after the second week and his throat was so burned. He doesn't remember cursing his doctor, but he said his doctor was right in describing how painful his throat burn could be during treatment, but he still appreciated his honesty.

Before Frank started his treatments, his insurance immediately approved payment. Frank told me:

> *"I had immediately been put in touch with the nurse case manager for Blue Choice, who was assigned to our company. She got it approved almost right away. Nurse case managers can really help patients through this process."*

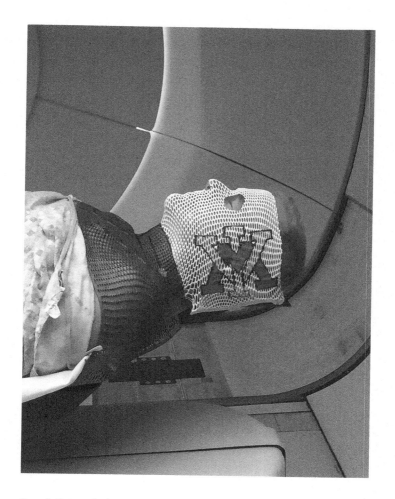

Frank Rosenthal receiving proton radiation at MPTC.

Keelin McGee will never forget her first appointment with her radiation oncologist:

> *"My initial consult was at Cincinnati Children's. I met with my radiation oncologist, and the head of lymphoma, Dr. O'Brien. I'll never forget her kindness. She set aside*

nearly an hour of her time to speak with my mom and me, answered all our questions, and she asked us questions we never thought of at the time. At a point in my treatment where I was fearful of receiving radiation, she calmed my fears and instilled every confidence within me."

Kate Weissman, who was treated at Mass General Francis H. Burr Proton Therapy Center in Boston, felt prepared for her treatments:

> *"All of my doctors were extremely transparent about the process of proton beam therapy; it was good because of that! I always knew what to expect and when to expect it, no surprises."*

For the past two years, I've been a board member and former co-chair of the Global Patient and Family Advisory Board at The Beryl Institute.

In these roles, I've liaised and collaborated on initiatives centered on the patient experience led by Jason Wolf, PhD, CPXP, and CEO of The Beryl Institute. Jason's unwavering commitment to elevating the patient experience is impressive. He has dedicated his life to it.

When I interviewed Jason about the patient experience, he reflected on the three key themes in his report and global survey on The Diagnostic Experience and what matters most to patients:

> *"The data revealed communication scored highest in importance, with 83 percent identifying its importance to*

the greatest extent. These include, **care team and the doctor provides information in a clear and understandable way, communication was shared in a compassionate and understandable way, and the care team and doctor takes the time to actively listen and address my expectations.***"*

Luckily and gratefully, once all the patients I spoke to were in treatment, I heard the most positive comments about the patient experience in line with the survey results and Jason's sentiments.

For my first appointment at MPTC, I met with Dr. Eblan as well as Dr. Chhabra, who at the time was completing his proton therapy fellowship at MPTC. Dr. Chhabra explained the mapping process where I would have a CT scan and the technicians would pinpoint the treatment area with tattoos so they would know where to send the proton beam when I was in treatment.

Dr. Chhabra created a memorable patient experience for me. I remember how intently he listened to my questions and seemed to read between the lines of my message. I don't know how he could do that so easily. I'd never met him before that appointment.

Even after my initial consult with Dr. Eblan, I had more questions for both doctors. Dr. Chhabra had a keen sense that I seemed scared to receive radiation treatment. He's truly gifted in making patients feel at ease. He creates the environment for patients to speak up.

In my appointment with Dr. Chhabra, my questions were primarily centered on my fitness goals. I wanted to stay active, not be sidelined from the gym as I had been after my mastectomy. Dr. Chhabra and Dr. Eblan focused on what was important to me. They were so patient with me and didn't make me feel stupid for being so scared.

I'm so grateful for their care.

During my interviews I asked some of the physicians:

How do you create the best patient experience for the patients you treat?

Arpit Chhabra, MD, Radiation Oncologist, Director of Education now at the New York Proton Center said:

> *"Well I like to think about it from the lens that the patient is driving this car. We are sitting in the passenger seat as physicians, telling them which direction to take; take a right, take a left, go straight, but ultimately, the driver is the patient and the patient has the right to decide what is best for them, play an active role in making the appropriate decision with respect to what is going to be the best for their trip/plan of care. So, I think the patient is the driver and I tell every single patient that I see my role as giving them direction and an understanding of what we think is best for them. But they've got the steering wheel in their hands. So, they should decide how they want to proceed."*

I couldn't agree more. At the end of my appointment, I felt reassured with my plan of care. I was ready to start treatment—ready to drive my car.

Carl Rossi, MD, Radiation Oncologist, Medical Director at the California Protons Cancer Therapy Center answered the same question:

"I think the experience starts at the point of contact with the center, when the patient first calls to inquire about getting scheduled for consultation. The individual whom they talk with has an especially important role in making sure the patient feels their case is important, their information will be collected in a timely fashion, and there will also be timely follow up for scheduling appointments. This continues at the time of consultation. I think the best thing I can do is pay attention to people and let them know [that] their case, while it may be common and typical in terms of a common diagnosis like prostate cancer, [is] still unique to them and spending a reasonable amount of time with the patient at first consult, I usually budget an hour. This also continues during the daily treatments when the technologists who interact with the patients the most and treat them as individuals and not just as a cog in the daily wheel."

I had so many memorable, compassionate patient experiences through my cancer journey. So many stand out—from my oncologist, breast surgeon, plastic surgeon, physical therapist, radiation oncologist, radiation therapists, and nursing teams. I can't thank them enough for healing me and bringing me through the journey to the other side.

Last, the nurse who held my hand when I went under anesthesia for my mastectomy was incredible. It was my first surgery ever, let alone two in one day. She was my angel before I went to sleep. I was so scared, but she held my hand and even squeezed it a bit and told me, "You will be okay."

The little things matter. I can still feel her hand on mine and remember those words, three years later.

PART TWO:
PATIENT STORIES

PROTONS & BREAST CANCER

MY STORY

"We do a good job of curing cancer, and adults are living normal lives. Yet, cancer recurrence or second cancers are devastating. They're difficult to treat. They have all sorts of horrible consequences, and they're not that unusual because people are living longer."

—CARL ROSSI, MD, RADIATION ONCOLOGIST, MEDICAL DIRECTOR, CALIFORNIA PROTONS CANCER THERAPY CENTER

Through social media, women have asked me specifically about proton radiation for breast cancer. Patients are asking the same questions I did three years ago, so not much has changed. The three most common questions are:

Should I consider proton radiation for my breast cancer?

Will insurance pay for my treatment?

My insurance declined proton radiation, what should I do?

Because of my own experience with protons and breast cancer, I knew I needed to write a specific chapter about it, and decided to start with my story.

Looking back, from the second mammogram, biopsy, and my diagnosis, everything was overwhelming. I'm an organized person and like to be prepared. Yet, I kept feeling like each time I had an appointment, I was unprepared.

The truth is, I wasn't prepared because I hadn't been through breast cancer before. So, I relied on my college roommate Annie, and my friends Nura, Kathy, and Karen. Each had a different diagnosis and plan, but Annie's was the closest to mine. We were diagnosed four years apart and, except for our cancer stages, we had the same diagnosis—even the tumor located in the 11:00 o'clock position for each of us. I learned early on that my breast became a clock for tumor placement, which was so surreal.

In January of 2018, after getting called back for a second mammogram, the technician said:

"Do you know why you are here?"

I said, "Yes, to get more images you needed."

She said, "Step into the machine and hold your breath."

So, I thought I must have moved the first time and they didn't get the right pictures. After she took the pictures, she came back to set up the next picture with me and said, as cold as ice:

"You have a mass on your left breast and we need to take more images. After we do that, you will go back to the waiting room and then come back for an ultrasound when you are called. We need to get more images so stay in your medical gown."

Then she stepped away and told me to hold my breath for the next image. But suddenly it sank in, and I said, "Wait a minute! What is a mass? Is it cancer? How big is it?"

I thought about a grape, a lemon, a golf ball, and I was scared out of my mind.

She said, "I can't tell you anything, now hold your breath for the last picture."

As I write, I can still hear her words and lack of empathy. I felt like I was at a fast food restaurant—a transaction—just another woman who might have breast cancer; she sees it all the time, next patient.

In the waiting room, women were wearing their patient gowns, patiently reading their phones and books while waiting to get called back for their mammogram. I felt like I was in outer space. I had just been to the gynecologist five months before I had this mammogram, and no lumps were found during my exam.

I texted my husband.

"The technician said I have a mass on my left breast! I'm so scared. I need to go back for an ultrasound."

Patrick said, "I'm coming back there right now."

I told him he couldn't, but by the time I got called back for the ultrasound, the technician said Patrick could accompany me. I asked the next technician about the mass. She told me they just needed more images and then I started to cry. She gave me a hug and then Patrick arrived in the room.

She took the images, and the radiologist came back in the exam room after she viewed my scans. She showed me and Patrick the area of concern. My husband asked what the chances were that I had breast cancer. She said it was "low, about 25 percent." I took a deep breath. Then she told me she wanted me to get a biopsy the next day.

Inside, I prayed I'd be in the 75 percent group.

My gynecologist ordered the biopsy, and I went at 7:30 a.m. the next day. By this time, my gynecologist referred me to a breast surgeon. It was the breast surgeon's nurse who I'd never met who called me back after worrying all weekend and the next few days, and she said, "You have cancer, but you have the good kind if you had to have it." I was shaking. I ran downstairs to tell Patrick I had cancer.

About a week later, when I had my appointment with the breast surgeon, who wasn't the surgeon that operated on me for different reasons, she recommended chemotherapy as the first step in my treatment, even before surgery. I learned this process is referred to as neoadjuvant chemotherapy. It's the reverse of adjunct chemotherapy, given to patients after surgery. Each patient's case is different, and the surgeon thought it was a tossup and said my oncologist would make the final call for my chemotherapy plan.

Later that same day, at my first appointment with my oncologist Dr. Harnden, I remember walking into her waiting room and feeling I was in a movie. It was surreal and sad. Some of the patients looked so sick-yet I had no symptoms and had cancer. Dr. Harnden reviewed different chemotherapy options with me. She ultimately recommended against neo-adjuvant chemotherapy. She wanted me to have the mastectomy first and then send my breast tissue to the lab to get an Oncotype score.

Dr. Harnden educated me about the Oncotype DX Breast Recurrence Score test and process. She explained that after surgery my pathology from my lymph node would be sent to a lab in California and the Oncotype score would be assessed. According to the Oncotype DX website, the lab would review the genetic makeup of my cancer "to determine how my tumor might behave in the future, including how likely it is to grow and spread or whether it is likely to respond to chemotherapy in addition to hormonal therapy."

Dr. Harnden spent a long time reviewing why she made this recommendation. It all boiled down to the risk of the cancer coming back and whether chemotherapy would help or potentially harm me. Cancer that comes back anywhere in the body is known as a cancer recurrence. If having cancer isn't bad enough, most of us learn along the way that cancer can come back not just in the breast but, as Dr. Harnden said, "I want to protect it coming back to your bones, liver, and brain." Wow, so much to learn about breast cancer.

The Oncotype score would give me a recurrence score (RS). At the time, a score under ten meant I wouldn't need chemotherapy, as chemotherapy could do more damage than good. Three years later and after multiple studies, a score of 1–17 versus 1–10 now means "a patient can potentially avoid chemotherapy" according to oncotypeiq.com

After my appointment with Dr. Harnden, I reached out to my village of family and friends and prayed for a score under ten (which meant my tumor was stupid, not smart, and not able to quickly multiply). Although I had other factors I still worry about from time to time, like a high amount of estrogen and progesterone in my tumor as well as a high KI-67 score which determines how quickly the cancer was multiplying, I prayed for a dumb tumor for a few weeks until my score came back.

I'm spending so much time talking about chemo here because we spent so much time thinking about chemo, praying I wouldn't need it. Radiation wasn't on the radar because cancer wasn't detected in my lymph nodes on the MRI prior to surgery.

From January 2018 to March 2018, I had a lot of appointments, prayers, and conversations about breast cancer. The first major step in getting rid of the cancer came on March 6, 2018, the day I had my mastectomy with Kirsten Edmiston, MD, Breast Surgery, and reconstruction that same day with Ariel N. Rad, MD, PhD at Sherber + Rad.

After surgery, as planned, my pathology was sent to the lab. When Dr. Edmiston called me a few days after surgery and told me I needed radiation, I was shocked. This wasn't supposed to happen. Ugh, they'd found more cancer in my lymph node that wasn't caught on the MRI!

Naturally, all sorts of thoughts went running through my mind.

Did the cancer move to my lymph node after the MRI so it wasn't detected?

Surgery was scheduled a month after the MRI, so then I thought maybe the cancer was running all around my body by then, yikes!

Other thoughts came to mind, will my breast implant explode from the radiation?

Will the radiation be more toxic due to my implant?

The more I thought, the more I concluded:

Maybe I should get the implant out?

I thought about so many crazy things. Thank goodness Dr. Rad helped me through my anxiety, as he told me it wouldn't be necessary to remove the implant. He didn't make me feel stupid for asking this question. We discussed the risk of radiation with my implant, and I remember him telling me about something called capsular contraction and I started worrying this would happen to me because of radiation.

Dr. Rad told me capsular contraction happens when the tissue becomes dense and hard in the implant capsule, where the implant sits, and it's a risk no matter the type of radiation. The capsule tightens and seemingly it feels like it's squeezing the implant. It's painful and can also cause the breast to move up on a patient's body. Although the risk was high, Dr. Rad said, "We are going to think positively that this isn't going to happen to you and think that you will be in the 60 percent of people that this doesn't happen to, not the 40 percent." Dr. Rad helped me shift my thoughts and I prayed for a new number.

I worked so hard to stay positive, prayerful, faithful, yet at night, at the gym, or during quiet times, my thoughts ran away from me. My family and friends helped me so much with positive affirmations and cheerful texts, emails, and phone calls.

I remained grateful that cancer didn't spread to more lymph nodes. Things could have been worse, and I looked on the bright side as much as I could.

After digesting the news and making plans for my first radiation consult, I went back into business mode—set appointments and did what I was told: work, get to the gym, and limit research!

When I learned about proton radiation through my husband's friend Jason, most people I talked to didn't know much about it. So, I called a friend in Boston who is a general surgeon. Dr. Val helped me understand the differences between photon and proton radiation. He explained that proton targets the treated area and stops at the treated site. In other words, the radiation wouldn't pass through my body he said. Since I had left-sided breast cancer and my tumor was in the 11:00 o'clock position, (inner chest wall) he thought it was reasonable that I ask for a consultation for proton radiation.

In the same breadth he said there weren't a lot of published clinical studies on proton radiation for breast cancer, but if it were him, he would want to protect his heart and lungs as much as possible to prevent complications and cancer recurrence in the years ahead. And he wanted me to do the same.

Three weeks after surgery, I had my first consultation with a radiation oncologist. He reviewed **photon** radiation and explained the breath hold technique, Respiratory Deep Inspiration Breath Hold (DIBH), which is a technique that requires patients to hold their breath for twenty seconds so that it will limit the amount of radiation exposure to the heart according to Stonybrook Caner Center.

The radiation oncologist was compassionate and explained the potential side effects of radiation therapy: skin burn, fatigue, skin discoloration, and change in implant size. He also heard I wasn't having chemotherapy. He thought Dr. Harnden told me, but she hadn't because my next appointment with her was in a few days. It was at this appointment that I heard my Oncotype score was under ten! My prayers had been answered.

My husband and I asked the radiation oncologist about proton therapy. We were told that it might be an option based on my mapping appointment where I would practice my breath hold and the technicians would map out my radiation plan and place removable tattoos on the radiation treatment area. Yet deep down, we knew we had to get another opinion for protons.

Days later I had my first consultation with Dr. Eblan and he asked me a lot of questions. He spoke to me about my clinical history and explained the differences between proton radiation and photon radiation (IMRT). I asked Dr. Eblan so many questions that he spent about over an hour with me and Patrick. He was so patient and caring. I think he knew how I worried I was.

At the visit, Dr. Eblan prescribed twenty-eight rounds of proton therapy. I would start treatment at the Maryland Proton Treatment Center (MPTC) as soon as I was able to lift my arms above my head which is difficult to do after a mastectomy but that's the position breast cancer patients hold when undergoing radiation. I also needed insurance to approve payment for the treatment.

It was in these first appointments and thereafter that I felt so grateful to be in Dr. Eblan's care. He listens with intent. To this day, I feel like he is sincerely partnering in my care.

As we worked through insurance denials and delays in radiation treatment, one day on the phone I asked Dr. Eblan what extracapsular extension meant in the lymph node. He told me extracapsular extension refers to the lymph node and he explained the lymph node is like a grape in shape. When a patient has extracapsular extension, it means the cancer is in the grape and breaks through the skin of the grape.

I wondered where the cancer went after breaking through the lymph node or the skin of the grape. Did the cancer stop travelling from there?

When I heard about this, it made me nervous but at least I knew what these terms meant.

I also decided it was time to research more about radiation, so I went to the American Cancer Society website, a place Dr. Harnden told me I should go for reliable and evidenced based information. There I found:

"Radiation for breast cancer patients is determined by whether a patient had a mastectomy, or breast-conserving surgery (BCS) like a lumpectomy and whether lymph nodes are involved."

I wanted to know more about the lymph nodes and why radiation was prescribed. I learned that the lymphatic system among its main duties protects the body from enemies such as bacteria, viruses, parasites, and fungi. It also removes and transports waste product and abnormal cells, like cancer cells from the lymphatic fluid.

Because of my lymph node involvement, I needed to have radiation to treat the other lymph nodes located in my arm pit, chest wall, clavicle, and the left side of my neck because if the cancer travelled, it would most likely travel there next.

I looked for studies and articles specifically about breast cancer and proton radiation, and our friend Dr. Val was right—there weren't a lot of studies published on the subject at the time.

I visited breastcancer.org and didn't find a lot of information there either. By this time insurance had declined coverage for my treatments, so I went to the chat room at breastcancer.org and asked if anyone had been treated with protons and approved for treatment by UnitedHealthcare. A few ladies responded. One was treated in the Midwest and others said insurance declined their treatments and they couldn't pay out of pocket, so they didn't get treated with protons.

Three years later, in 2021, women are still asking how they can get insurance to pay for proton radiation in the breastcancer.org site. Other women are commenting on their suggestions. This is so disappointing and sad to me, yet this is the inspiration for my book!

When I interviewed the radiation oncologists, I asked a few of the doctors about proton radiation specifically for breast cancer.

Dr. Rossi of the California Protons Cancer Therapy Center discussed the evolution of proton radiation in breast cancer, saying:

"Up until about a decade ago, a physician couldn't easily do whole breast treatment, and definitely could not do peripheral lymphatics. So, we started protons on patients who are candidates for partial breast radiation, or in some cases, depending on anatomy, whole breast radiation. But those patients can also be treated with X-ray therapy (photons).

"But what's changed over the years is the deployment of the Pencil Beam scanning system which allows us to treat very large, very irregular shapes. So, suddenly, the ability to treat the whole breast and the lymph nodes in the center of the chest and the lymph nodes in the axilla, becomes feasible with protons. And if you're looking at left sided breast cancer, in many cases, you will markedly reduce the radiation dose to the heart over anything you could do with X-rays. This is true in general, in protons, anytime. When the fields become larger and more irregularly shaped, there's greater and greater disparity in normal tissue dose between protons and X-rays. So, the breast cancer we treat here, many of them are locally advanced and if you try to do that with X-rays, you can, it's tough. We're able to do that same thing without putting nearly as much radiation in the heart, and it's clear that radiating the heart, like radiating most normal tissues, is not something you want to do unless you absolutely have to.

"I think there is a lot to know, and that people need to realize there is still a lot we are learning about the use of protons in breast cancer. It is certainly not required for every breast cancer case. Protons appear to be most beneficial in those individuals who have left breast tumors that also required treatment of regional lymph nodes, particularly those in the center of the chest. This is not to say they are not beneficial in other circumstances, but this one patient group that appears to benefit the most in terms of reducing heart and lung radiation dose. By the same token there are many patients in with a comparative plan of protons versus X-rays (comparing proton to photon) that showed little if any difference in radiation dose to underlying lung and heart. So, in essence it often comes down to the individual's anatomy and tumor location."

A study that was recently published from the Danish Breast Cooperative Group showed that the risk of cardiac events begins within five years after patients finished radiation versus historically a major chronic cardiac event didn't occur until well after ten years. From the study:

"Over the past fifteen years, evidence has accumulated that radiotherapy for breast cancer can increase the risk of subsequent heart disease. The increase in risk per gray (the way the does is measured) of mean heart dose was 19 percent for patients with photon-techniques where data were available for precise dose estimation."

Protecting my heart was one of the reasons I was prescribed proton therapy for my case. When I saw the images of the heart being partially exposed to radiation with photons versus protons, I was relieved this treatment was prescribed for me.

And J. Isabelle Choi, MD, Radiation Oncologist, Director of Research, Clinical Director, New York Proton Center also has a view that aligns with Dr. Rossi's sentiments about cancer recurrences and the potential of minimizing this impact from proton radiation:

"We are achieving superior disease control and long-term survival in multiple cancer types. But what that also means is that patients are now living long enough more often to develop recurrences of their cancer. For example, in breast cancer, given our now excellent clinical outcomes in a large subset of these patients, we are now seeing more late recurrences that occur ten to twenty years after their initial cancer treatments.

Previously, we would not necessarily see these patients back for these recurrences due to more limited survival. Many of these patients received radiation therapy for their initial breast cancer presentation but also require radiation again for their recurrence. This is very difficult to do safely and well with photon radiation due to concern for excess toxicity to the tissues already irradiated the first time, such as the heart and lungs. Proton therapy provides these patients with a safe and effective opportunity for a second cure as it can allow for sparing of the important organs from receiving more radiation dose while still fully treating the area of recurrence."

After my radiation treatments, people reached out to ask me what it was like.

I've heard the ads that tout that proton treatment is painless and for the most part that's true.

Yet, on my first day and on most of my days, there was one single dose that seemed to hit me like a lightning bolt as I've mentioned. By the second week of treatment, I could almost time when that happened. It was painful; no one could explain it.

By the second to last week of treatment I had severe burns. I was given the option to stop treatment in the last week, but as painful as it was, I kept going. I needed to get to the finish line and ring that bell! I focused on being Boston Strong. I thought about when I ran the 2001 marathon, and thought this can't be as painful but, toward the end, it was worse.

Yet, I stayed positive and kept a smile on my face. I knew that I needed to do that, otherwise it would consume me even more than it already had. I just wanted to get through. I didn't want to be glum or sad, I just needed to keep going.

Patients who I've met since treatment also ask questions about which lotions I used during treatment. I didn't like the lotions that were given to me at the treatment center. The Miaderm and other lotions stung my skin. Instead, I asked Dr. Eblan if I could use something else. He told me I could but there were no studies on what could or couldn't happen to me based on the change in lotions. I was okay with that and felt like Dr. Eblan was truly partnering with me in my care. If I used the alternative lotion at night instead of in the morning before treatment, he said I could try other lotions.

I settled on coconut oil after experimenting with olive oil, emu oil, and other oils that I mixed. I found that Spectrum coconut oil, either at Whole Foods or Amazon, soothed my skin. I also wonder if the coconut oil is why my skin didn't turn brown after treatment. Maybe a study on different lotions during treatment would be helpful for patients. I've recommended coconut oil to other patients who've also checked with their doctors and found it equally as helpful.

After I was severely burned, nothing helped the pain on my skin, only time. The burn felt like I was rolling around in broken glass.

As predicted by my nurse and Dr. Eblan, the burn got worse after treatment. I couldn't imagine it could be worse, but it was. I saw Dr. Eblan a week out from treatment and he prescribed Silvadene for the burn. I used that for a short time, and within roughly four weeks of treatment, my skin started making a big turn for the better.

I also found it difficult to wear a bra during radiation. It's so embarrassing even writing this, but after I found True & Co bras, at Nordstrom I felt a lot more comfortable. Many Nordstrom stores have sales associates that are trained and certified in breast cancer bra fittings before surgery and after. My salesperson was a saint, an angel to me. She called me a beautiful lady when I felt so burned and ugly. It's the little things that go such a long way.

I never lost my appetite and ate most of what I would normally eat, however my nutritionist told me to include more protein in my diet to help my skin heal. I incorporated more fish, and, in my mind, I was doing what I could to heal. I also practiced intermittent fasting, something I learned from Dr. Harnden. This seemed to really help boost my energy level.

I worked out at the gym through the entire treatment. It was my way of feeling normal, on my routine, my old self. I couldn't lift heavy weights but that was a small price to pay.

Toward the end of my treatments and thereafter, I felt dizzy and lightheaded. I thought it was from the pain from the burn. I spoke up when I was at my follow up appointments and my doctors thought I was dehydrated and encouraged me to drink more water.

I wasn't getting better so my nutritionist asked me to get my get bloodwork done to see why I was so lightheaded. It turns out I was drinking too much water and my sodium levels were very low. She recommended that I take Nuun tablets in my water each day and I felt almost immediately better. It truly takes a village as my symptoms presented the same as dehydration, so it was easy to mistake one for the other.

Facts about proton radiation and breast cancer are encouraging from different proton center websites in the United States.

THE UNIVERSITY OF TEXAS MD ANDERSON CANCER CENTER

"Proton therapy may be especially beneficial for breast cancer patients by minimizing damage to nearby tissue and critical organs such as the heart and lungs."

CALIFORNIA PROTONS CANCER THERAPY CENTER SAN DIEGO

"Studies have found that proton therapy for breast cancer provides better coverage of the lymph nodes, while substantially reducing average radiation doses to the heart and lungs. This ultimately results in a reduced risk of cardiac events, lung cancer and pneumonitis."

UF HEALTH FLORIDA PROTON THERAPY INSTITUTE

"When the amount of radiation to the heart and lungs is decreased, so is the risk of developing side effects such as heart disease, reduced lung function, or secondary cancer."

When Dr. Eblan and I talked about protons and breast cancer, he weighed in on the same themes Dr. Rossi and Dr. Choi discussed:

"What is the cost of heart damage or a secondary cancer twenty years from now? As physicians, we're thinking about those issues all the time when treating patients. And thinking about the benefits but also the potential downsides of radiation often can drive our decision to seek proton therapy because we're worried about these future risks to the patient."

What is the benefit of protons? It's the potential to preserve quality of life, the ability to work and be self-sufficient, and to minimize the risk of secondary cancers later in life.

I don't think insurance companies should make the decision for access to protons, our physicians should.

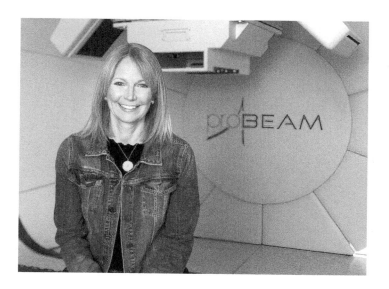

That's me at MPTC 21 months after treatments ended under the Varian ProBeam machine.

PROTONS & BREAST CANCER

JILLIAN'S STORY

"Patients should think about their bodies. If something is wrong, despite a doctor dismissing it, keep pushing as patients know their bodies the best. Pay attention to that inner voice telling you something is wrong."

—JILLIAN BENSTEIN, CANCER SURVIVOR

Patients I've met have asked me if I've heard of anyone who had breast cancer on the right side and had proton radiation that insurance approved—meet Jillian Benstein.

Jillian, a thirty-eight-year-old instructional designer working in the greater Washington, DC area, intuitively knew something wasn't right. She was busy living her life with her family and working full time. She didn't feel an obvious lump like a pea or a marble, but her right breast didn't feel as smooth as normal.

She was concerned because her mother and grandmother suffered through breast cancer, but when examined, her medical team dismissed it as just being fibrosis breast tissue. They felt she didn't need a mammogram and reminded Jillian insurance would not pay for it as she was under forty. This didn't sit right with Jillian. She called the doctor's office back and explained she would pay out of pocket if she had to, but she couldn't ignore it. She's glad she did.

After her mammogram, Jillian was sent for a biopsy of a suspicious area. When the biopsy came back, Jillian was diagnosed with Stage IIB invasive lobular carcinoma (ILC). According to the American Cancer Society, it's a challenging cancer because the cancer starts in the lobules (milk glands) and spreads to surrounding tissue. Because of the location of the cancer, sometimes it's hard to detect on a mammogram or during a self-exam. Both ILC and IDC can metastasize to other parts of the body.

After her diagnosis, in November of 2018 Jillian's doctor found something in her other breast and wanted to do a biopsy. Jillian declined the additional biopsy and decided to have a double mastectomy, the removal of both breasts. Later she had reconstructive surgery.

Like me, after her surgery she found out the cancer had spread to her lymph nodes. By January of 2019, she started a heavy dose of chemotherapy, with sixteen infusions over five months of time.

After all she'd been through, Jillian was concerned about having radiation. She asked her doctor:

"Is there a better option for me?"

Jillian decided to see another oncologist for a second opinion. In this appointment, Mei Firestone, MD, mentioned proton radiation, and she was sent for a consultation with my radiation oncologist, Dr. Eblan.

Dr. Eblan educated Jillian and me on proton radiation and informed each of us about a clinical trial that would measure the efficacy of proton versus photon treatment for breast cancer. Once Jillian learned about proton therapy through Dr. Eblan's consultation, like me, she knew protons were right for her.

Dr. Eblan prescribed proton treatment as the best option for Jillian's cancer but warned her it might be a struggle to get her insurance to approve it. Like me, Jillian also had UnitedHealthcare. She also enrolled in a clinical trial. Dr. Eblan prepared his letter for insurance to approve. Like other patients, Jillian was also turned down by her insurance provider not once but twice. Again, Dr. Eblan had to prepare another letter of medical necessity.

In the meantime, Jillian reached out to me through my website Proton Radiation Buddy. She was frustrated that her insurance declined authorization for protons and wanted to advocate for herself. I introduced Jillian to Kate Weissman, a fellow proton advocate at the Alliance for Proton Therapy Access. Kate spoke to Jillian and encouraged her to share her story with the Alliance.

On August 6, 2019, Jillian sent me an email that read:

"Oh my goodness, they approved it! I am still having a hard time believing it's true. I haven't talked to Dr. Eblan yet, so I still feel like they made a mistake or something. I'm feeling *so* grateful! Thank you so much for fighting to get yours approved. I know everyone who pushes back helps to build a wall for insurance."

I was so happy for Jillian. I also thought deep down, since her breast cancer was on the right side, I wasn't sure which way her case would go. After hearing other patients lose their cases, I prayed Jillian's would be approved.

During our interview in the fall of 2020, we reminisced on her experience with protons. Like the other patients in this book, I asked Jillian:

What should a patient know about proton radiation?

Here are Jillian's thoughts below:

- Proton exists.
- Insurance will give you a struggle.
- Clinical trials *might* help you get a foot in the door with insurance.
- There needs to be more proton centers built to offer services to more people.
- Proton covers a lot more cancers than I thought.
- The state of Maryland is cost neutral, so photon and proton treatments cost the same.
- Side effects are minimized with protons.
- Protons reduce the damage to healthy tissue and organs.
- Challenge your radiation oncologist if they don't offer protons. If you don't ask, you won't know what might be right for you.

- Don't underestimate the time it takes for insurance to approve or deny treatment.
- Sometimes patients' skin won't look the same after treatment but the long-term effects of protons versus photons is worth it.
- It was recommended I have physical therapy to help with long term mobility effects of the radiation. I think this made a big difference for me and, if anything, I wish I started sooner.
- About five weeks into treatment my skin became raw, inflamed, and started to peel. However, I was aware this was a side effect of any type of radiation.

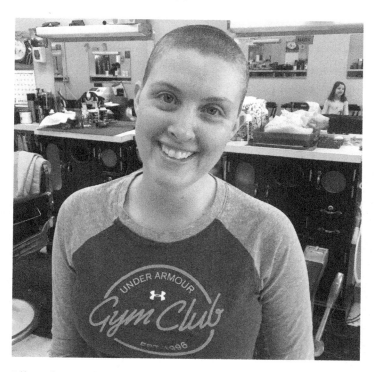

Jillian during chemotherapy treatments.

I also received similar recommendations for physical therapy (PT), but my breast surgeon recommended I go to PT before and after proton radiation. I agree with Jillian, it made a big difference. It was through my experience with my physical therapist Caitlin that I was diagnosed with lymphedema, a condition which can occur after the lymph nodes are removed during breast cancer surgery. I was fitted with a lymphedema sleeve, and would see Caitlin for lymphatic massage and therapy to move my lymphatic fluid through my body, which is important for healing.

Like me, Jillian was also so appreciative of Dr. Eblan's care and persistence with our insurance providers.

I was so happy to share Jillian's story. She's incredibly strong, upbeat, and wants to share her story to help others, especially since her breast cancer was on the right side. She's doing well post treatment and is so grateful for proton treatment and the impact it had on her health and wellbeing.

PROTONS & BREAST CANCER

MARIAM'S STORY

"While cancer interrupted my senior year of college at UC Santa Barbara, my insurer's actions caused me the most stress."

—MARIAM TARIQ, CANCER SURVIVOR

I met Mariam through the Alliance for Proton Therapy Access. Here's Mariam's story.

In December of 2016 at twenty years old and a junior at University of California Santa Barbara (UCSB), Mariam Tariq felt a lump in her breast. She wasn't sure what it was, so she called her pediatrician. Her doctor told her if the lump moved around, and it didn't hurt, then it probably wasn't anything to worry about. Mariam was relieved.

In June of 2017 she felt the lump had grown. She talked to a coworker whose mom had the BRCA gene and a history of breast cancer. The coworker told Mariam because of her mom's genetics, she'd been through an ultrasound and biopsy. She said it was easy to do and encouraged Mariam to get checked out.

Back at home in Irvine, California, Mariam went to her doctor who sent her for an ultrasound and biopsy of her breast. She was leaving for New York the next week to visit family and celebrate Eid, the end of Ramadan, so she was grateful to be seen right away. She had both tests and didn't think twice about it.

Mariam was eating in a restaurant enjoying her second day in the Big Apple when she received a call from her doctor.

Miriam told me, "She dropped the news: the biopsy was cancer. And just like that, my whole world was shaken."

At twenty-one years old going into her senior year at UCSB, Mariam was diagnosed with breast cancer.

Mariam thought:

"Okay, how are we going to do this? I'm in New York on vacation and I live in Irvine, California and now I have breast cancer."

When Mariam finished the dreaded phone call and heard of her diagnosis, her cousin got things moving. She booked an appointment for Mariam at Memorial Sloan Kettering Cancer Center in New York City. The doctors there read her pathology and diagnosed her with Stage III HER2-positive breast cancer.

According to breastcancer.org, Stage III breast cancer means the cancer has moved beyond the breast, may have invaded the lymph nodes, but hasn't invaded other organs. Depending on the tumor(s) size, amount of lymph nodes involved, or no lymph nodes will determine the level of the stage—IIIA, IIIB, or IIIC. Each patient's case is unique to their own pathology, tumor size, and lymph node involvement, as well as how many lymph nodes were invaded.

In Healthline.com's article "Chemotherapy and Targeted Therapy for HER2-Positive Breast Cancer," when breast cancer is HER2-positive like Mariam's, it means the cancer cells make too much HER2 protein, which can cause tumors to grow more rapidly than with other forms of breast cancer.

In about one of every five breast cancers, the cancer cells have extra copies of the gene that makes the HER2 protein. HER2-positive breast cancers tend to be more aggressive than other types of breast cancer, according to the Mayo Clinic.

After her doctor discussed her diagnosis and pathology, she was sent for a positron emission tomography (PET) scan, which the Mayo Clinic defines as a scan which uses a radioactive tracer and can sometimes detect disease before it shows up on other imaging tests. Mariam's scan didn't detect additional disease in her body-her cancer hadn't spread.

Timing was on Mariam's side. Two new drugs were just released, Trastuzumab (Herceptin) and Pertuzumab (Perjeta). These drugs were used in chemotherapy to treat Mariam's HER2-positive breast cancer. The drugs drastically improved the diagnosis and the prognosis for treatment and eased Mariam's worries.

As luck and good karma would have it, her doctors in New York knew a former colleague that had just moved to LA. So, Mariam was referred to a new oncologist, Heather L. McArthur, MD, PhD, Medical Director at Cedars Sinai Hospital in LA. Mariam flew back to Irvine and was seen for an appointment the very next day.

Because Mariam had a family history of cancer, during her first appointment, the oncologist discussed the importance of genetic testing. At a young age, Mariam's brother had passed away from cancer. She also had others in her family, including relatives in Pakistan, with a history of breast cancer.

Mariam's genetic tests came back with the TP53 mutation, which is referred to as Li-Fraumeni Syndrome.

According to an article on Ambry Genetic's website called "Understanding your TP53 Genetic Test Result," everyone has two copies of the TP53 gene inherited from each birth parent. Mutations in one copy of the gene can increase a person's risk of certain types of cancer such as soft tissue sarcoma, osteosarcoma, female breast cancer, brain tumors, adrenocortical carcinoma (ACC), leukemia, and potentially other types of cancer. Those with this gene mutation may have a lifetime risk, more than 90 percent.

Because of the TP53 mutation, Dr. McArthur recommended a double mastectomy. Mariam would have six months of chemotherapy, a double mastectomy, and then proton radiation treatment. Like me, Mariam didn't know there was a difference between different types of radiation:

"I didn't even know what proton was, and I couldn't differentiate between proton and photon because they sound so much alike. My doctor said I should get proton for three reasons: my lymph nodes were positive, I'm young, and finally proton radiation would decrease my lifetime risk of secondary cancers."

Dr. McCarthur referred Mariam to Catheryn M. Yashar, MD, Radiation Oncologist at California Protons Cancer Therapy Center. As soon as Mariam met with her doctor, the team at California Protons Center submitted her case for prior authorization approval. Then they scheduled Mariam for her mapping simulation, which is needed prior to treatments.

As part of the simulation, according to OncoLink, a patient has a CT scan to pinpoint the exact location for radiation treatment. This treatment area is referred to as the "map," which determines the specific radiation plan for the patient. Tattoos are placed on the treatment area to outline the map for treatment.

As Mariam began the simulation process, she got a call from the financial department at California Protons:

"We don't want to worry you but, UnitedHealthcare denied your claim for treatment, and we're going to fight it, but we just wanted to let you know."

Mariam easily recalls this conversation like most of us who have experienced it:

"It freaked me out because I thought no one seems to know about proton radiation, there are only a few centers around the world. How much is this going to cost if I don't get it approved? I didn't even think of the financial repercussions until that very moment. I started thinking about my parents going into medical debt over my treatment. It was so stressful."

At this point in Mariam's journey, she understood the benefits and differences of proton versus photon radiation to treat her breast cancer. She didn't want to be treated with photon radiation. With her family's support and the support of the team at California Protons, she continued to appeal the denials from UnitedHealthcare.

Mariam started twenty-eight days of radiation treatment **without** insurance approval. Her parents told Mariam they would figure things out with the medical bills if insurance didn't approve her treatments.

She was a senior in college then, and each day she drove herself to and from treatments. When back in Irvine, she kept up with classes, not wanting to miss out on her senior year. Mariam is such an inspiration!

In the background, California Protons continued to appeal her case. Mariam reflected on how supportive they were in her fight for her own insurance coverage. As Mariam was in treatment, she would hear:

"Yes, you were denied again but we are submitting another appeal so we will let you know."

At some point, the only option left for the team at the California Protons Therapy Center was to appeal to the California Insurance Commissioner. The team at the center asked Mariam if she wanted to keep fighting for her insurance coverage and approach the Commissioner. She agreed.

In the meantime, Mariam got in touch with the Alliance for Proton Therapy Access. The Alliance helps patients like Mariam have a voice through their contacts in the media and their understanding of the challenges of the insurance system. Mariam spoke to Molly Daniels, the Executive Director at the Alliance. Molly asked Mariam if she wanted her plight with protons and insurance to go to public. Molly offered to share Mariam's story with the media to educate the public on the behind-the-scenes insurance process which happens every day.

Mariam didn't know what to expect. Like me, she felt called to act in some way:

> *"I figured if it would be helpful for other people who are trapped in the same predicament, then I should tell my story."*

Then she got the call from California Protons Cancer Therapy Center:

> *"UnitedHealthcare overturned your case."*

Later she received the formal letter from UnitedHealthcare stating her case was overturned. She saved the letter and the letter from the California insurance commissioner.

Many of us who have been through the prior authorization insurance denial and appeal circle of failure look back at these approval letters as a sign of gratitude to our physicians and finance teams, a sign of perseverance and strength for all of us involved in the process.

For those of us who have gone through the complicated and stressful process and had our cases overturned, it feels like winning the toughest sports game with no preparation. While we waited for cancer treatments or as they got started like in Mariam's case, we kept going. We gutted it out until the clock ran out. Except this isn't a game. This is cancer care.

When Mariam went public with her story, the media picked it up. In June of 2018, one of the doctors on her team, Parag Sanghvi, MD, Radiation Oncologist at the California Protons Cancer Therapy Center was interviewed by ABC 10 News San Diego. In his conversation with the reporter, Dr. Sanghvi said:

"When patients have this particular genetic mutation, we do everything possible to avoid radiation as we know radiation can also cause secondary cancers. Proton beam therapy was the safest in her case."

The insurance provider, UnitedHealthcare, told ABC 10 News San Diego:

"A radiation oncologist reviewed the case and said other types of radiation would be an equally effective treatment for Mariam's condition."

Mariam also spoke out through her own blog which was featured in *The Santa Barbara Independent*:

> "At the heart of my insurance fight was proton beam therapy. My doctors ruled out traditional radiation treatment as too risky because of a genetic susceptibility to secondary cancers. Proton therapy's precision would target my tumor and minimize radiation exposure to healthy tissues, significantly reducing my risk of secondary cancer. It was a no-brainer to everyone but UnitedHealthcare."

Mariam started proton radiation in April of 2018 and completed treatment in May of 2018.

Her proton treatments were approved by UnitedHealthcare in October of 2018.

Mariam, Jillian, and I were all diagnosed with breast cancer. We had different diagnoses within breast cancer but coincidentally we were all customers of UnitedHealthcare. Although we most likely had different health plans within UnitedHealthcare, we all went through a similar process: breast cancer diagnosis, prior authorization request, denial, appeal, denial, appeal, and so on.

All of our cases were overturned by UnitedHealthcare.

I have often wondered if insurance companies believe we will just give up, stop the fight for what's best for us as there's other types of radiation that insurance will approve. Not in my case, but in many cases the proton treatment costs more money than photon radiation, so maybe that's why insurance won't approve it, despite doctor's orders.

I couldn't find studies that determined whether breast cancer patients abandoned treatment due to insurance denials, but I found a recent study from July of 2019. MD Anderson reviewed 903 head and neck patients seeking proton therapy treatment and reported 19 percent of patients abandoned treatment while waiting for insurance to approve or deny treatment as prior authorization delays resulted in up to four months of delayed treatments.

I also wonder if insurance companies think about secondary cancers as a result of radiation? It turns out there's a lot of literature on this topic. In fact, I Googled "Does radiation cause secondary cancers?" and within 0.49 seconds I had 54,500,000 articles!

The first listing, "Second Cancers Related to Treatment" by the American Cancer Society states the risk of cancers from radiation with most of these cancers occurring after ten years of radiation. Variables affecting this risk include age, dose of radiation, and area treated.

Secondary cancers from radiation are scary! It's something many cancer survivors think about when our bodies don't feel quite right.

It makes me think: Is an insurance company's decision on approving coverage for treatment plans a short-term decision? Because I can't help but wonder: What is the downstream economic impact on the insurance company's bottom line profit if a customer is diagnosed with cancer again in ten years? I don't know the answer.

One thing is certain: UnitedHealthcare is making good money, as most companies in a capitalist society aim to do.

According to United Health Group's 2018 annual report, the year Mariam and I were treated:

Revenues came in at "$183.5 billion, which grew by $20.2 billion over 2017 revenues."

I'm not suggesting the government control these decisions versus the market forces of competition in a free market such as capitalism. I'm simply asking how much is too much? Especially when people's health and wellbeing are at stake.

Three years after treatment, Mariam is doing well! She's enjoying roller skating under the sunny skies of southern California. She's passionate about social justice issues, and currently works for Mayor Farrah Kahn in the city of Irvine, California.

Mariam's story is another illustration of not giving up and thus seeing her case overturned!

PROTONS &
HEAD & NECK CANCER

COACH RON RIVERA'S STORY

"One day after beating the Dallas Cowboys, Washington Football Team Head Coach Ron Rivera took another victory lap, but this lap celebrated a different win: the end of his cancer treatments."

—ESPN SPORTS

I interviewed Head Coach Ron Rivera in the winter of 2021. Here's Coach's story.

In July of 2020, just before the start of the NFL season, Head Coach Ron Rivera of the Washington Football Team felt a lump in his neck. He was on his way to a two-week vacation and just thought maybe his glands were swollen. But when he got back, he asked the team doctor, M. Anthony Casolaro, MD, to check it out.

Dr. Casolaro felt the lump and told Coach Rivera he would keep an eye on it and see him in a week. A week went by and Dr. Casolaro reexamined Coach Rivera and decided to send him for an MRI. The radiologist read his scan and decided to send him for a biopsy of his lymph node. The biopsy confirmed squamous cell carcinoma.

Because the biopsy was positive, Coach Rivera was sent for another biopsy four days later to determine if the cancer was viral. During this appointment, Coach Rivera's second biopsy confirmed the cancer was viral.

In a matter of minutes, Coach Ron Rivera's life and schedule was upended.

According to Stanford Health Care, squamous cells line the outside of many body organs, including the mouth, nose, skin, throat, and lungs. Cancer can start in the squamous cells and then spread to the lymph nodes in the neck or around the collarbone.

At the early stages of a cancer diagnosis, patients move quickly from one appointment to the next to gather all the necessary facts to determine the course of treatment. As part of the multi-disciplinary approach, Coach Rivera's next appointment was with Patty Lee, MD, Ear, Nose, and Throat (ENT) specialist. Dr. Lee performed an endoscopy to determine the point of origin. Coach Rivera's wife Stephanie Rivera joined Coach for the appointment.

Ahead of this appointment, Coach Rivera heard a lot of positive feedback about Dr. Lee, and he quickly learned why:

"She was tremendous. She was excellent and she has the best bedside manner."

Like Coach Rivera, most of us who are diagnosed with cancer aren't prepared for what's coming. I said to family and friends, "I don't have a playbook running through my mind as to what to do next like I do at work." As patients, in a moment's notice we build trust and go with the doctor's game plan without preparation or an understanding of this game we're hoping to win.

So when Dr. Casolaro and Washington Football Team owner Mr. Daniel Snyder suggested proton radiation as a consideration for cancer treatments, Coach Rivera knew this was something to take seriously as a treatment option. Both Dr. Casolaro and Mr. Snyder were familiar with the benefits of proton radiation versus traditional photon radiation for Coach Rivera's diagnosis. In Coach Rivera's words:

"Dr. Casolaro and Daniel Snyder talked about proton radiation with me and said, 'You should try and get proton radiation.'"

Advocating for Coach Rivera's health became top priority for Dr. Casolaro. He attended Coach Rivera's first appointment with Gopal K. Bajaj, MD, MBA, Radiation Oncologist; President, Radiation Oncology Associates, PC. Dr. Casolaro continued to stay involved in Coach Rivera's medical discussions and treatment plans.

Ultimately, Dr. Bajaj recommended proton radiation as it would minimize damage to healthy tissues in Coach Rivera's throat as the proton beam stops at the target and doesn't pass through the body like photon radiation would.

Dr. Bajaj submitted Coach Rivera's case for insurance approval.

Coach Rivera's insurance declined coverage for proton radiation.

As quickly as his insurance company declined payment for his treatments, Mr. Snyder stepped in to advocate with Dr. Bajaj, as did John F. Deeken, MD, Medical Oncology. Each made phone calls to the insurance company on behalf of Coach Rivera.

Within the same day, his case was overturned.

It was during this moment, Coach Rivera re-affirmed: all patients need an advocate. Someone to help speak up on a patient's behalf. Someone willing to fight insurance if needed. It doesn't matter who you are, everyone needs an advocate.

As Coach Rivera progressed through his appointments and treatment plan, he learned he needed chemotherapy at the same time he received proton radiation, so before his treatments started, he needed to visit an oncology dentist.

Seeing an oncology dentist is part of the protocol for head and neck cancers according to Jack Martin, DDS, Chief of the Section of Oncologic Dentistry and Prosthodontics, Department of Head and Neck Surgery at the University of Texas MD Anderson Cancer Center:

"A dental examination before radiation for head and neck cancer is important for two reasons: to impress on the patient the need for fluoride therapy and to remove any restorable, abscessed, or periodontal-diseased teeth in the field of radiation therapy."

After the appointment with the oncology dentist, he was cleared to begin his cancer treatments.

Coach Rivera wanted to start his treatments right away before the start of the 2020 NFL season. Along his journey of appointments, he heard positive feedback about proton radiation treatment:

> "You know, when I asked the doctors, 'What should I do?' They all said, 'We think you should do proton therapy.' So, as far as I was concerned, photon radiation was out of the question."

As luck would have it, after the first week of treatment, the proton machine went out of service for a few days. To keep Coach Rivera's treatments going, he had photon radiation.

He told me about the differences between the two:

"I got two days of photon treatment, and I could tell the difference. My salivary glands just went berserk. I kept spitting. I mean, constantly spitting, because my salivary glands were inflamed and just kept producing saliva for about a week before they finally settled down. For a week and a half, I had cups in my house in my car and my office everywhere from two treatments of photon. I didn't realize how much it affects you when you get the broad X-ray beam with photon as opposed to the pinpointed beam in proton. That was probably the biggest lesson I learned about the differences between photons and protons."

As his cancer treatments progressed into the fall of 2020, Coach Rivera continued to coach the Washington Football Team. It was his first season coaching in Washington, DC. He didn't miss a game. Everyone was in awe of his strength and determination; a cancer survivor or not, a football fan or not, Coach Rivera set the example for resilience and perseverance. Not only was he beating cancer and staying strong, but his team also rallied behind him wearing "Rivera Strong" t-shirts; they played one of the best NFL seasons the city had seen in a long time. As a cancer survivor and a Washingtonian, I'm so proud of our city's head coach. He set the example and then some.

On Monday morning October 5, 2020, Robin Roberts, also a cancer survivor, interviewed Coach Rivera on the *Good Morning America Show.* Coach Rivera had just coached a game against the Baltimore Ravens the day before. As Roberts began telling Coach Rivera's story, she reported he would receive two bags of IV fluid on the sidelines to stay hydrated throughout the game. She asked him how and why he continued to coach while receiving radiation and chemotherapy treatments. He responded:

> *"The doctors said it was important to keep as much of my routine as possible and then listen to my body when I needed rest. I thought if RGB (Ruth Bader Ginsberg)*

can do it, so can I. People are watching me. I want to set an example."

During his interview with Roberts, he was vocal about access to healthcare for all. We talked about it, too. It's a travesty that the United States spends more on healthcare than any other country and has worse outcomes. According to a study by the Commonwealth Foundation published in January of 2020:

> *"While the United States spends more on health care than any other country, we are not achieving comparable performance...the United States healthcare system is not doing its part. Our analysis shows the United States has the highest rates of avoidable mortality because of people **not** receiving **timely,** high-quality care."*

One of the reasons people have not received timely care for services is due to the insurance providers prior authorization process which slows down timely treatment, tests, and necessary care.

During our interview, Coach Rivera connected to this pain point in the insurance process through his mom's sister who passed away from a heart condition she had twenty-nine years ago:

"She received a very minimal remedy for it, and then twenty-five years later, as an adult, she had issues and she passed away. But before my mom had gotten a chance to take her to see her own cardiologist, her cardiologist looked at her sister's records and basically said, 'You know, apparently, about twenty-five years ago, she didn't have the right insurance, because this was how they treated it. If they had done this, she wouldn't have this issue today.'"

It's sad and disappointing to hear this tragic story as a result of not having the proper healthcare coverage.

So I asked Coach Rivera, what should we do?

We both agreed our legislators can help with policy that prohibits insurance delays due to the prior authorization process.

For example, the American Medical Association (AMA) started a grass roots effort called #FixPriorAuth to do just that. Since January of 2017, the AMA has been advocating for prior authorization reform which would improve access to healthcare. According to their survey of one thousand physicians:

- Ninety-one percent reported prior authorizations have a negative impact on patient clinical outcomes.
- Ninety-one percent said prior authorization delayed patients' access to necessary care.
- Eighty-eight percent of physicians reported this problem has gotten worse in the past five years.
- Every week a medical practice completes roughly thirty-one prior authorization requests, which take the equivalent of 14.9 hours of physician staff time to complete.

In January of 2021, the Center for Medicare and Medicaid Services (CMS) seemingly rushed a ruling on prior authorization. An article in Radiology Business outlined:

"CMS issued a final ruling aimed at easing the burden of onerous prior authorization policies on both patients and providers. Advocates in the physician and payer communities meanwhile believe the policy will do little to fix the problem."

Although this is a first step to creating electronic prior authorizations versus sending these authorizations by fax and phone, it only applies to Medicaid, the Children's Health Insurance Program (CHIP), and qualified plans on federally facilitated exchanges. How disappointing; as Medical Group Management Association Anders Gilberg, Senior Vice President of Government Affairs, issued in a press release on January 15, 2021:

> "MGMA views this final rule as a huge, missed opportunity to address prior authorization, the top administrative burden facing the nation's medical group practices. The rule will do little to address widespread health plan abuses that delay and deny patient care. This failure will require practices to continue deploying multiple, manual prior authorization workflows, including using phone, fax, and payer web portals."

According to the ruling, insurers have up to three days to answer to an "urgent" prior authorization and seven calendar days for "non- urgent" requests.

Waiting three days for an urgent medical need is daunting, unacceptable, and not just for cancer patients, but for all patients seeking care.

On October 26, 2020, Coach Rivera rang the Hope Bell. He finished seven weeks of proton radiation and concurrent chemotherapy treatments. Again, through it all, Coach Rivera continued to coach. He didn't miss a game. He's truly an inspiration.

During his experience from diagnosis to the bell ringing ceremony signifying the end of his proton and chemotherapy treatments, Coach Rivera felt he had advocates in Dr. Bajaj and Dr. Casolaro.

As we reflected on Coach Rivera's cancer journey, I couldn't help but reflect on my own and those who've shared their stories in this book in an effort to try to help others. The shared experiences of a cancer diagnosis, treatment, and crossing into the end zone of recovery and survivorship is a humbling experience as Coach Rivera explained:

"When those radiation technicians come in and get each person from the waiting room and I watched those people go back for treatment, they were from all walks of life, we just waited our turn. No one is treated specially or differently while you're getting your treatment. It is very humbling. It put a lot of things into perspective again. So, I was very fortunate, but I didn't know any better. I was pushing for my treatment; I want to get it done. Let's go. Let's get this out of me. But, again, I'm fortunate because of who I am, I guess. But I just think that's wrong."

Now, Coach Rivera is passionate about advocating for access *and* timely access to healthcare including access to proton therapy. He's grateful for his family, the Washington Football

Team organization, friends, fans, and the entire medical team throughout his journey. He's doing well post-treatment and is looking forward to his second year as the Head Coach of the Washington Football Team.

As Coach Rivera mentioned, he had advocates that quickly jumped in, recommended proton therapy, and helped him get his case for insurance approval overturned **in the same day**. It's amazing to me Coach Rivera's case was also denied on the first try. The pattern of automatic denial seemingly applies no matter who the patient is. Yet, Coach Rivera was the only patient I interviewed whose case was overturned on the same day. Thank you to Coach Rivera for wanting to make a difference through sharing his experience.

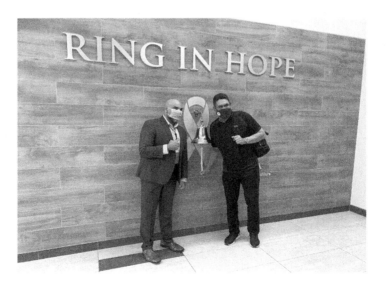

Coach Rivera ringing the Hope Bell with Dr. Bajaj.

PROTONS & HEAD
& NECK CANCER

BRIAN'S STORY

"I'm thankful I found proton treatment through my own research, but it's an immoral crime it isn't a covered treatment by Independent Insurance Association (IPA's) and some insurances."

—BRIAN HINDS, CANCER SURVIVOR

I met Brian and his fiancée Julianne Boardman in 2020 when I committed to publishing a book on proton radiation. Through social media chat groups related to cancer, I announced:

"I'm publishing a book on proton radiation. Do you want to tell your story?"

Julianne responded almost immediately. She and Brian were in a fight with their insurance provider right as I asked the question.

Meet Julianne's fiancée, Brian Hinds.

Brian, fifty-two, is an amateur herpetologist and VP of Operations at an internet provider and lives in La Verne, California. In 2020, he noticed a swelling in the left part of his neck. He'd been traveling in the mountains the previous weeks and thought he might have an infection.

He went to his primary care physician who examined him and told him he was not alarmed and sent him to an ENT physician for follow up. Brian saw the ENT, who examined him and looked down his throat with a scope. She stated bluntly, "I have good news and bad news. You have tonsillar cancer, but the good news is: You can beat this."

According to Cancer.net, in 2019, head and neck cancers account for about 4 percent or 65,630 of total cancer diagnosis in the United States. In general, there are three main types of treatment for head and neck cancer: surgery, chemotherapy, and radiation. The diagnosis, stage, and other factors, such as the location of the cancer, determines the treatment plan of whether to use one, two, or all these treatment options.

When Brian found out he needed radiation, he started researching his options on his own. His ENT didn't refer Brian for proton treatment. But he was curious what would happen to his body during radiation treatment.

Brian thoroughly reviewed studies on protons versus photons for head and neck cancers. He and Julianne quickly realized the significant difference in side effects to healthy tissues and structures while in radiation treatment and thereafter.

One of the studies Brian and Julianne reviewed by Blanchard et al. examined patients with oropharyngeal carcinoma, which includes the tonsils, soft palate, and base of the tongue, and is a type of head and neck cancer. The goal was to understand the differences in outcomes between intensity-modulated proton therapy (IMPT), also known as Pencil Beam scanning, and photon radiation, using intensity-modulated radiotherapy (IMRT) and delivering photon radiation at different angles using advanced computer programming to deliver the treatment.

The study ran from 2010–2014 with an average patient age of fifty-eight. The study consisted of fifty patients who received IMPT to one hundred patients who received IMRT treatments.

Among the study's conclusions:

> *"Patients who received IMPT had a reduced rate of feeding tube usage and dependency, a side effect known to occur with IMRT."*

Being diagnosed with cancer is tough enough. Losing or restricting the ability to eat and drink is a potential side effect with IMRT. In addition, cough and controlling saliva is also a side effect that can be very challenging to manage. These side effects can significantly impact a patient's quality of life, even alter the ability to talk. This was important for Brian and Julianne. It would have been for me too!

In other areas of research for head and neck cancer, in *the International Journal of Particle Therapy*, researchers sought to analyze the national trends and disparities for patients seeking proton therapy for head and neck cancer. The study begins with the differences in IMRT versus proton for head and neck cancers. It explained the implementation of IMRT has been shown to decrease both acute and chronic side effects. However, adjacent healthy structures can still receive considerable radiation doses with IMRT because of the physical properties of the photon beams.

From all the literature, Brian knew proton radiation would be a better treatment option with less toxicity to his surrounding tissues and structures. He would also expect less short- and long-term side effects. His quality of life mattered, and it mattered for every patient I interviewed.

After discussing the pros and cons of IMPT and IMRT, in September of 2020 Brian requested that his physician place a prior authorization and referral to the California Protons Cancer Therapy Center in San Diego, California. Toward the end of October, his treating physician let him know that she could not request authorization, nor could she make the referral to the California Protons Cancer Therapy Center as the medical director of the IPA informed her this was not allowed under the guiding principles in the IPA. She stated the only care authorized was IMRT within their IPA healthcare system.

According to the American Academy of Family Physicians, IPAs follow a set of "Guiding Principles." The first of the eight guiding principles:

"IPAs should organize a health care delivery system which produces optimal health outcomes for patients."

How do the guiding principles align with optimal health outcomes? Maybe the first guiding principle should clarify optimal health outcomes is defined by the type of plan a patient has at the time of treatment.

Because the IPA could not make the referral to California Protons Cancer Therapy Center, the center would not be able to submit claims to Brian's IPA-HMO. So, Brian scheduled a self-referred consultation appointment with Ryan Grover, MD, Radiation Oncologist, Department Chief at the California Protons Cancer Therapy Center. Dr. Grover has been working for over fifteen years treating thousands of patients with proton radiation.

Once Brian's treatment plan was created, a group of his professional associates and family members organized a GoFundMe account to help him pay for protons. In mid-November 2020, within two weeks after his consultation, he began proton treatment at California Protons Cancer Therapy Center.

Knowing Brian's insurance would be coming up for yearly open enrollment, Julianne began researching which insurance companies under a PPO plan paid for proton therapy in previous years. As a result, in December Brian was able to change to a PPO plan under Blue Cross, and after a month of requests for authorizations, denials, appeals, and additional information requests to the California Protons Business office, Blue Cross finally authorized treatment halfway through his treatment plan. Of course, everything prior to

December would not be covered by Blue Cross, so he still had over $47,000 worth of out-of-pocket expenses.

Despite this being a relief, the entire process caused so much stress for Brian and Julianne during a time that is difficult for all cancer patients facing cancer treatments.

Ironically, for twenty-five years Julianne has been a certified medical assistant in Los Angeles, California. In her role in various doctors' offices, she's been working on behalf of thousands of patients seeking prior authorization approvals for various medical services and treatments, advocating on the patient's behalf. Since 2017, she became a certified professional coder working in coding and billing. She knows the process inside and out. Brian and Julianne shared their advice for some patients use protons for benign tumors:

- Be your best advocate, and fight for what is your right as a patient. Fight for your care.
- Prior to a patient requesting an authorization from their insurance company, contact the insurance company and request a complete copy of coverage details. Specifically, carefully read the cancer treatment guidelines including radiation, chemotherapy, radiology, infusion therapy, etc. Be well informed on how the insurance company has written their guidelines for treatment and the appeals processes, and follow the guidelines.
- Allow the proton center to request the initial authorization and, if denied, allow them to appeal the denial. At this point, the patient can file their own appeal and the appeals process should be followed as per the insurance company's guidelines.

- Do not request a verbal appeal from the insurance company. Everything must be in writing. Anything shared verbally must also be included in written communication.
- Receiving an approval for a consultation does not automatically indicate proton therapy treatment is approved by the insurance provider.
- Ensure no steps in the appeals process are bypassed by the patient or the insurance company.
- Patients have the right to ask for the rationale used by the health insurer to determine a denial of coverage. Request this in writing so you can base your appeal on the information given from the insurance company.
- Continue to follow-up with the health insurer through all levels of appeal, even if continued denials are received.
- If all levels of appeal are still denied, speak with the proton therapy center's financial counselor or billing representative about the following options:
  - Requesting an independent review board review the case.
  - Filing a complaint with the state insurance commissioner.
  - Hiring an attorney.
  - Contacting the local state representative or senator who may have influence with some insurance companies.

Brian's proton treatments ended on January 11, 2021, when Brian rang the Hope Bell. It was difficult to eat solid foods right after treatment, which can happen from proton radiation, too. But a few weeks later Brian was enjoying solid foods again and is now on the road to a better quality of life after proton radiation.

When I first met Brian and Julianne in the fall of 2020, I shared in their anger and frustration. I felt the same way in 2018 when I went through the same experience with United-Healthcare. As patients and caregivers, we believe through sharing our stories, we will show others fighting for proton radiation treatment that the fight might be the best thing they've ever fought for.

PROTONS & PROSTATE CANCER

JOHN'S STORY

"I had forty-four proton treatments. My insurance declined coverage, but the team at the Maryland Proton Treatment Center (MPTC) appealed my case, they worked it out, somehow, they ended up approving my case and insurance paid for my treatment. I didn't hear much about it, it was handled, and I could focus on treatments."

—REVEREND JOHN CRESTWELL, CANCER SURVIVOR

Forty-nine-year-old Reverend John T. Crestwell, Jr is African American and a Minister at UU Church of Annapolis. On June 28, 2018, he was preparing the eulogy for a member of his congregation who was murdered in a mass shooting in Annapolis. Five people were killed in the attack on the offices of the *Capital Gazette* newspaper.

I met John through the team at MPTC. I reached out to interview him and hear his story with proton radiation. During our interview, John said, "It was a very stressful time." Suddenly the local and national media descended on Annapolis at a time of deep sadness and mourning throughout the community and within his congregation. Over one thousand people were expected to attend the service, including the governor's wife and other dignitaries who wanted to pay their respects for the five who lost their life.

John vividly described to me:

> "And then no sooner than I put my eulogy to rest, I got the phone call. My doctor said to call him right back. And I thought, oh shit. He told me right then, when I called him back, I have prostate cancer, but they caught it early."

There were three spots of cancer on John's prostate, which is a gland located below the bladder, and the cancer starts in the cells of the prostate gland.

John told me:

> "And I just couldn't believe it, would not believe it. And I didn't feel my greatest, but I thought I was just stressed out because one of my members just got murdered by a crazy man."

So, amid preparing for this important service, John needed to go through the first steps in his cancer journey. He took off the month of July to go to appointments and research what he should do next.

Like John, I also wanted to research the different treatment options for breast cancer, but there weren't many places to go at the time.

One of the first steps in any cancer diagnosis is determining the location of the cancer, the size of the tumor, the stage, and grade of the cancer. Through these initial discussions with the doctor, patients begin to learn more about their body—more than they ever knew before.

In Bob Marckini's book *You Can Beat Prostate Cancer: And You Don't Need Surgery to Do It,* he educates patients on what the grade of cancer means. Specifically, it "describes how closely the individual cancer cells resemble normal cells of the same type which is an indication of how fast the cancer is growing." The stage "describes the extent of the cancer in a patient's body, or how far the cancer has spread."

From my own research on prostate cancer, I found the most widely used system to determine staging in prostate cancer is from the American Joint Committee on Cancer (AJCC) which uses the TNM system. The TNM system is based on five pieces of information which include the characteristics of the tumor, lymph node involvement, whether the cancer has spread (M for metastatic), the PSA level at the time of diagnosis, and the grade group which is based on the Gleason score.

According to the American Cancer Society, PSA stands for Prostate Specific Antigen. Men who have a level between four and ten have about a one in four chance of having prostate cancer. If the PSA is more than ten, the chance of having prostate cancer is over 50 percent. John's PSA was 5.2.

There is so much known about cancer but not actually what causes each person to be diagnosed. So that's why cancer is described in terms of risk factors. From the American Cancer Society, prostate cancer risk includes:

- Age, which is the most common risk factor. The older a man, his risk for prostate cancer increases.
- Other risk factors include geography, ethnicity, family history, gene changes, smoking, and other factors.

As John researched his options, he scheduled an appointment at MPTC and learned more about the different treatment choices he faced. After his appointment his options were:

- Proton radiation: which would require forty-four treatments and lots of time off from work to travel to and from the proton center which was roughly thirty-five miles from where he lived.
- Traditional radiation: photon radiation.
- Surgery to remove the cancer.
- Brachytherapy, which is a procedure that places radioactive sources within the treated area of the prostate to kill the cancer while healthy tissue receives a minimum dose of radiation.

Together with his wife and doctor at MPTC, John chose proton radiation because as far as he was concerned, this was the least invasive and the best treatment to manage side effects. He wanted to maintain the best quality of life he could and be fulfilled by being in service to others.

As John began his treatment, he experienced a few blessings; as he described:

"I had a religious awakening. During this period of time, I was doing a lot of studying and reading about religion. I felt this energy surge in my body and I was thinking what is wrong with me? Am I dying? What is going on? I started connecting different religions together and seeing mathematics and sounds and I could just connect everything for a moment."

John also experienced healing while under treatment, but not just for his prostate. He said:

"After two treatments, my hip totally loosened up. The proton beam was shooting right at my hip which had bothered me for years. Eventually my hip tightened up again, but not the way it was. And it was aching every day when I slept at night. And after two treatments, it literally went away."

John asked me if I also experienced side effects from protons. I said "yes" and described the swelling and pain in my chest wall area and told John about my fractured ribs. John said protons must have been "frying my bones." Fractured ribs aren't common from proton radiation and we chatted about what I could have potentially faced with photons. Who knows?

John had minimal side effects from treatment, which included fatigue during and after treatment. Almost three years later, John is doing great! His current PSA is 1.05, where previously it was 5.2. He continues to serve his parish and enjoys time with his wife. Here's his advice on prostate cancer treatments:

"Proton radiation is the least invasive option that I know of to kill cancer with minimal side effects. I'm living a healthy life and feel great."

I've had patients reach out to me who have been newly diagnosed with prostate cancer. Not knowing if they would need radiation treatment, I refer them to Bob Marckini's book as it's the best resource for prostate patients, written by a patient. It helps patients understand prostate cancer and their options for treatment, including proton radiation. I'm grateful to have met John and heard his story of faith and triumph over prostate cancer through his treatments with proton radiation.

PROTONS & PROSTATE CANCER

JIM'S STORY

"Insurance wasn't going to sway their hard-headed opinion that proton therapy was not a coverable treatment."

—JIM GRUNERT, CANCER SURVIVOR

Jim and I met in 2020 through the MPTC alumni group. We follow MPTC through social media, and I posted a question in our chat group:

"I'm publishing a book on proton radiation, does anyone want to tell their story?"

Meet Jim Grunert.

At fifty-eight, as a healthy human resources professional who lived in a suburb of Rochester, New York, Jim knew the importance of scheduling his annual physical appointments. In 2016 after a routine physical, his primary care physician (PCP) discovered an elevated PSA. His PCP prescribed an antibiotic for a potential infection called prostatitis. Jim would remain on this antibiotic for several weeks and then have his PSA retested.

It was during this second round of bloodwork Jim's PSA had elevated to an eight. As previously mentioned, men who have a PSA between four and ten have a one in four chance of having prostate cancer. Jim's PCP told him he would need to see the urologist.

Jim met with the urologist who recommended a biopsy and on July 29, 2016, he had fourteen to sixteen pieces of his prostate biopsied. Jim won't forget how he felt. It wasn't fun, to say the least. He scheduled a follow up appointment on August 18, 2016, with his doctor to review the results.

Jim feared the worst as he waited for the biopsy results. During this time, he researched prostate cancer and found out there are false positives with the PSA. According to the Mayo Clinic:

"The PSA test can detect high levels of PSA that may indicate the presence of prostate cancer. However, many other conditions, such as an enlarged or inflamed prostate, can also increase PSA levels. Therefore, determining what a high PSA score means can be complicated."

Yet, after the biopsy, Jim started to experience blood in his urine. Jim called the doctor on August 8 to relay his symptoms. It was then his doctor told Jim the blood wasn't a problem, but that he did have prostate cancer and would discuss the results during the August 18 appointment. Jim was very upset when he heard the news, yet he carried on to his next appointments.

Jim met with his urologist to discuss the biopsy results. His doctor told him his prostate cancer was aggressive and diagnosed him with cT1, Gleason 8, large volume (enlarged), localized prostate cancer.

According to the American Cancer Society, the "cT" is the doctor's best estimate of the extent of a patients' disease based on a physical exam and a patient's biopsy. Since Jim's Gleason score was an eight, his cancer was characterized as "high grade."

Based on these results, Jim's doctor told him he needed surgery in addition to eight weeks of photon (IMRT) radiation. Jim's doctor explained the potential side effects of surgery and radiation, which consisted of urinary and fecal incontinence, impotence, and potential collateral damage to other organs as a result of radiation. His doctor said he was fairly young and he had a decent possibility of regaining an acceptable amount of his urinary and sexual health.

A study published in the NCI states incontinence is a "common postoperative complication in 50–90 percent of patients who undergo the operation. Erectile dysfunction may occur in 10–90 percent of patients who undergo surgery."

This didn't sit right with Jim.

The doctor recommended surgery the following month, but Jim told his doctor he needed time to wrap his head around the fact he had cancer. He wanted to use his annual vacation to Florida to let the diagnosis settle in and then he would rebook an appointment to discuss the next steps. Jim used this time in the Florida Keys to continue to research prostate cancer. He ordered a few books, including Robert Marckini's book *You Can Best Prostate Cancer: And You Don't Need Surgery to Do It.*

Jim scheduled a second opinion at Roswell Cancer Institute in Buffalo New York and after reading Robert Marckini's book, he also contacted Loma Linda University, The University of Florida Health Proton Therapy Institute (UF), and the Maryland Proton Treatment Center (MPTC). Markini's book was included in the packet from Loma Linda and UF, so Jim ended up with three copies!

MPTC was the first to respond to Jim's inquiry, so he decided to make an appointment at the center. Jim's insurance company at the time of diagnosis was MVP. They authorized the consultation at MPTC, but deep-down Jim knew they would potentially deny treatment coverage.

On October 5, Jim and his wife Alice flew from Rochester to Baltimore and visited MPTC. After Jim's consultation, he learned he was a good candidate for proton radiation. As he departed the center, he thought if insurance declined authorization for proton treatment, he would pay out of pocket. Jim was grateful for his employer who remained flexible to his work schedule throughout these treatment appointments.

Jim's second opinion on October 7 at Roswell Cancer Institute proved to be a bit more concerning. His physician told him he thought his cancer diagnosis was worse than the first urologist. His doctor agreed with the first doctor and said he would need surgery and photon (IMRT) radiation treatment.

However this doctor told Jim he was also a prostate cancer survivor. He said his prostate surgery had been performed by the first urologist who diagnosed Jim. Despite the fact this first surgeon was an excellent surgeon, this doctor had to wear a diaper due to urinary incontinence. It was then Jim decided he wanted to avoid surgery.

After a few more scheduled appointments, Jim scheduled his first of forty-four proton treatments on January 30, 2017.

Before Jim's treatments began, the doctor submitted his prior authorization to MVP to ask for coverage for the treatments. At this point it was December and they denied coverage. The holidays passed, and in January Jim's insurance changed to Excellus Blue Cross Blue Shield (BCBS). They also denied authorization and coverage for the treatment. Despite all the information on efficacy, better patient outcomes, and the fact that proton and photon treatments cost the same at MPTC, Excellus BCBS declined his treatment. Jim's physician appealed his case.

All along Jim was prepared to pay out of pocket, but who would want to do that? Not Jim or me or anyone I've met! But sometimes that's the decision patients must face. It seems so unjust.

Many of us patients wouldn't even think to ask what percentage of time insurance might overturn a case. So, I researched to find out how often this happens inside and outside of cancer care.

I found a study cited by the California Nurses Association which stated that in 2016 in the state of California, 60–80 percent of insurance denials were overturned or reversed when taken to an *independent medical reviewer.*

Specifically:

- Sixty percent of cases insurers denied as "**not medically necessary**" were either overturned by California Department of Managed Healthcare (CDMCH) an independent medical review or ultimately reversed by the insurer.
- Eighty percent of cases insurers denied as "**experimental**" or "investigational" were overturned or reversed by the insurer.

As this study reveals, an independent medical review process is often triggered after a prior authorization is declined. Sometimes patients must file a grievance for denied coverage of a medical treatment, prescription, or diagnostic test and then wait for a third-party review to weigh in on the case.

Jim's treatment was denied again by Excellus BCBS while urgent attention and appeals letters were sent by the team at MPTC. Jim also wondered if a radiation oncologist had reviewed his case or not. Although Jim appealed his case with the support of his physicians, he needed to start treatment. Jim ultimately paid out of pocket for the entire treatment plan, but not everyone who needs radiation can do so after the peer-to-peer reviews fail to cover treatment.

Jim experienced the prior authorization, denial, appeal, and peer to peer review process, and it was a nightmare for him. Despite it all, Jim had a positive attitude. Like many of us who were treated at MPTC, the care, compassion, and sense of humor of the team goes a long way. It impacted my healing, and it did for Jim, too.

In the waiting room at MPTC, Jim got to know a lot of people, especially a few men who were also being treated for prostate cancer. Jim and all the gentlemen he met did so well with their proton treatments. They had minimal side effects and were able to enjoy a more normal life even as they received cancer treatments.

After daily treatments, Jim would join his new pack of friends and take bike rides or grab a beer within the Inner Harbor of Baltimore. One time after each of the guys finished treatments, they took a car ride through Little Italy, a quaint area of Baltimore full of shops and delicious Italian restaurants. Jim and his friends were in search of a certain bakery they'd heard about when suddenly at the same time they all had an urgent need to pee. They stopped the car and ran into a restaurant with one bathroom and one after another they took their turn. The restaurant owner didn't know what to expect, but graciously allowed the guys to take care of business. After the trip to the bathroom, the guys laughed and carried on with their day, enjoying time together in the city all the while undergoing cancer treatment.

The urgent sense to pee is a side effect of treatment since prostate patients follow a protocol of bladder control before and during treatment. They can also have inflammation in the area from the radiation.

To keep the prostate in a consistent position during treatments, prostate patients are instructed to have an empty bowel and a full bladder during treatment. This might sound easy but think about doing this multiple days in a row, as in Jim's case for forty-four days of treatment.

I remember on my first day of radiation treatment, I sat in the waiting room with all the patients and caregivers. A gentleman next to me was sipping a cup of water in his medical robe and I was in mine. He said I looked like I was new as he hadn't seen me before. I explained it was my first day of proton treatment. He asked me why I was being treated and I told him I was treated for breast cancer. He said, "Breast cancer patients have it so easy compared to prostate patients." I thought that was so interesting and strange to say to someone. Then I asked him what he meant by that, and he said, "We have to drink a few cups of water to keep our bladder full during treatment; you don't need to do that." He was right, I didn't need to do that. But breast cancer patients have to hold our arms over our heads during treatment, which can be difficult for some patients after a mastectomy.

After treatments, Jim and his buddies returned to the Hope Lodge where they stayed during their time in Baltimore. The Hope Lodge is a free "home away from home" for cancer patients and their caregivers, provided by The American Cancer Society. There are thirty Hope Lodges across the country, including Puerto Rico. Patients have access to the Lodge if they are in active cancer treatment and live more than forty miles away. Each offers a community of healing where guests can share a meal and get involved with activities at the Lodge or within the host city. Guests have access to a consistent list of amenities throughout each Lodge, including free transportation to and from treatment centers. The concierge at MPTC helps their patients arrange for lodging options, including The Hope Lodge in Baltimore.

Four years after treatments, Jim is doing great! He's living a healthy and happy life. Jim stays active, has great energy, and started playing pickleball. He volunteers for the Red Cross as a transportation specialist who picks up donated blood and brings it back to the central lab. He's also the chairman of the Town of Henrietta Planning Board which is in suburban Rochester, New York.

He enjoys being part of the growth and development of his town. Jim and Alice stay true to their annual trip to Florida in March where they relax and spend time on the beach.

Hearing Jim tell his story of prostate cancer, proton radiation, and the friendships he's made through cancer treatments was heartwarming. Jim and I felt that by talking about our stories with proton radiation we might be able help educate patients through our lived experiences.

Here is Jim's advice for patients seeking proton treatment for prostate cancer:

> *"I'd recommend patients research into all possible treatments. My urologist didn't provide me any options; he just told me he'd be doing surgery on me the following month. It was up to me to see if there were other choices and I eventually had to tell him no, I was not having surgery.*

"I would also recommend second opinions on diagnosis and biopsy results. I realize sometimes time is of the essence but in most cases prostate cancer is slow growing, so the patient has time to do their research."

I agree with Jim's advice for patients. It's so unfortunate Jim's case wasn't overturned, yet Jim was able to receive proton treatment by paying out of pocket. I'll cover more ways patients can advocate for themselves later in the book. But we've already learned through several of our patient stories, including my own, that getting a second opinion might be the best place to start to advocate for an alternative treatment.

PROTONS & PROSTATE CANCER

DAN'S STORY

"From Spartanburg, South Carolina to Charlotte, North Carolina, to Chattanooga, Tennessee, to London, England to Knoxville, Tennessee, I travelled a lot of miles to be treated with proton radiation for prostate cancer."

—DAN IVEY, CANCER SURVIVOR

I met Ginger Ivey through the Alliance for Proton Therapy Access Facebook group where people share stories, ask questions, and learn about proton therapy. These groups are great for people who will start treatment, are in treatment, and even after. Sometimes I've found other cancer related chat groups to be too much, but not this one.

Dan is a retired builder and Ginger is a family practice nurse. They live in Moore, South Carolina. From 2009 to 2015, Dan had an elevated PSA and nodule and had regular visits to his urologist who told Dan his nodule was a calcified hematoma (collection of calcified blood) outside the prostate, likely from a previous fall which caused a pelvic fracture.

Then in January of 2015, things drastically changed. Dan's PSA elevated, which caused Dan to seek a second opinion in Charlotte, North Carolina from Daniel L. Watson, MD, Co-Director, Presbyterian Robotics Institute, Chief of Urology, Presbyterian Hospital and Novant Southern Piedmont Region, Physician Director, Presbyterian Multi-Disciplinary Urology Oncology Clinic. Dr. Watson was recommended to Ginger by her colleague. Dr. Watson performed a biopsy and then, in March of 2015, Dan had a robotic assisted prostatectomy.

Within nine months of surgery, Dan's PSA elevated again. Both Dan and Ginger were concerned. After some research and through conversations, Dan and Ginger found Joseph J. Busch Jr., MD, an Oncological Radiologist who specializes in advanced prostate imaging at the Busch Center in Chattanooga, Tennessee. Dan and Ginger visited Dr. Busch four times, driving from Moore, South Carolina so Dan could have multiparametric MRI's. According to Rosenkrantz AB, Hemingway J, Hughes DR et al., this type of MRI is used for men at risk for prostate cancer and improves insight into the pathology of the diseased cells.

In September of 2019 during the fourth MRI, Dan's doctor found an area of concern in the right iliac area of his pelvis. At the time, Dr. Busch was going to London to do advanced imaging with Anwar Padhani, MBBS, FRCP, FRCR, Consultant, Radiologist and Professor, Cancer Imaging at the Paul Strickland Scanner Centre Mount Vernon Cancer Centre,

Northwood, UK. Ginger and Dan decided to travel with Dr. Busch so he could have a PMSA scan, which at the time wasn't approved by the FDA for prostate patients in the United States.

According to the FDA, a PMSA PET scan can more accurately detect prostate cancer cells in the body that may metastasize (spread) from the prostate. Since Dan's visit to the UK for the test, it's been approved for use by the FDA in December of 2020.

Dan also had a whole-body diffusion scan. From the GE Healthcare website, diffusion weighted imaging (DWI) is an MRI technique that can provide information about lesions and soft tissue structures. This unique way of imaging can find cancer and not expose patients like Dan to additional radiation from a CT or PET scan.

From the DWI, the doctor found a node in his right iliac area, so Dan was sent for proton therapy treatment back in the United States. Proton therapy could target the area while sparing healthy tissues and structures in the treated area.

South Carolina didn't have a proton center, so Ginger and Dan researched a few different proton centers they could drive to. They ultimately chose Ben Wilkinson, MD, Radiation Oncologist, Medical Director, Provision Healthcare in Knoxville, Tennessee, who was the closest and recommended by Dr. Busch.

Dr. Wilkinson prescribed thirty-three proton treatments over six weeks.

Since Dan had Medicare and AARP Plan F with United-Healthcare, his treatment was covered 100 percent with no delay in treatment.

After all Dan's been through, his insurance process went smoothly. When his doctor sent his case in for prior authorization, he was able to have his treatment paid for 100 percent by his insurance without delay. This is the way it should be! Through Dan's supplemental coverage through AARP and UnitedHealthcare, his treatment was covered.

At the same time, a patient's treatment shouldn't be delayed or declined and deemed experimental treatment just because the patient isn't on Medicare and AARP Plan F. This makes no sense and is so unjust to those on other plans, especially those covered by UnitedHealthcare.

All of us proton survivors are grateful when other patients' treatments are approved without delay.

I'm grateful Ginger was willing to share Dan's story so others could learn from his journey.

Two years post treatment and Dan's PSA is now 0.00–0.01. He's seen now by Daniel L. Watson, MD, Urologist in Charlotte, North Carolina, and every three months Dan also has telehealth visits with Dr. Wilkinson who's now located in Santa Maria, California.

Dan is doing well after treatments and is enjoying life in Moore, South Carolina with his wife Ginger.

Unfortunately, this quick approval for treatment may not be available to patients like Dan in the future due to pending legislation with the Radiation Oncology Alternative Payment Model (RO-APM) mentioned in the previous chapter. Dan was approved for proton radiation without delay due to his Medicare *and* AARP supplemental plan. If this new payment model is enacted in July of 2021, this could potentially prevent access to proton radiation for this patient population.

PROTONS & PEDIATRIC CANCER

NIKKI'S STORY

"They told us Nikki had about a thirty percent chance to live. Proton therapy saved Nikki's life."

—JERRY SCHINDLER, NIKKI'S DAD

In early 2021, my sister Robin's friend Sue Curtin emailed me and said she'd heard I was publishing a book on proton radiation. She told me about a strong young woman named Nikki Schindler who volunteers with her at the senior center. She wanted to introduce me to Nikki and her dad Jerry.

I immediately wrote back "yes!" I wanted to meet Nikki and her family. Jerry and I scheduled a time for all of us to talk in early February of 2021.

Here's Nikki's story.

In fifth grade and at the cusp of being ten years old, Nikki Schindler had really bad headaches. She sat in the back of the classroom, so her mom thought she might need glasses. Then one morning, Nikki's mom took her to the pediatrician.

He examined Nikki and noticed swelling behind her eyes. He had another doctor look, and he noticed the area was swollen, too. They sent Nikki to the neurologist that afternoon.

According to Nikki, the neurologist didn't notice anything that seemed "weird."

She walked and stood, and everything seemed fine, only to find out the next day that it wasn't. The doctor prescribed an MRI of the brain as the next step.

Nikki was sent to the South Shore Hospital Weymouth where she had an emergency brain MRI, and a brain tumor was found.

In Nikki's words:

> "We scheduled an MRI, but the MRI was a month out because everything was so backed up. But the next day there was a snowstorm. Everyone canceled their appointments. So, we took the first appointment in the morning because they had an opening. I went with my mom, who is a nurse. I had my MRI, and they had to use contrast and my mom knew that wasn't good. They told us that day I had a brain tumor."

On March 5, 2015, at ten years old, Nikki was diagnosed with aggressive medulloblastoma with metastasis within her brain. According to St. Jude's Hospital, this type of cancer starts in the region of the brain at the base of the skull. The tumors tend to spread to other parts of the brain and to the spinal cord.

Nikki didn't have the common symptoms like dizziness, nausea, and fainting. She had headaches off and on, and some of the headaches were debilitating just before she was diagnosed.

Nikki was immediately sent to Children's Hospital in Boston. At Children's Hospital, doctors gave her medicine for five days to reduce the swelling in the brain. On the fifth day doctors performed her craniotomy, which is a surgery that removes part of the bone from the skull to expose the brain for surgery. This is an intense surgery that opens the skull to be able to get at the area of the brain that needs to be treated. The surgery took twelve hours.

By the time of her surgery, Nikki's cancer had already metastasized to a different part of her brain. Nikki's doctors told her and her parents she needed to have six months of aggressive chemotherapy. Prior to that she needed to have thirty days of proton radiation.

Just like most of the patients I interviewed for this book, Nikki's parents had never heard of proton radiation. Most of us think radiation is radiation. It's not until patients like Nikki, me, and others are diagnosed that we find out about protons.

Nikki was sent to Massachusetts General Hospital's (MGH) Francis H. Burr Proton Therapy Center, the second proton center opened in the United States back in 2001.

Nikki's doctors explained there wasn't much more they could do as the tumor had really spread within her brain. Specifically, there was a section of the tumor that had grown into another area of the brain and they couldn't do another surgery in that area.

Boston Children's had already consulted with the doctors at MGH: David Ebb, MD, Pediatric Radiation Oncologist and Nancy Tarbell, MD, Pediatric Radiation Oncologist, Dean for Academic and Clinical Affairs and the C.C. Wang Professor of Radiation Oncology at Harvard Medical School.

Nikki's parents asked Dr. Tarbell if protons would save Nikki's life. Her doctor said:

"We wouldn't be treating Nikki if we didn't think we could save her life with protons."

According to Nikki's parents, Jerry and Maureen, Dr. Tarbell knew all of the studies on protons and she treated Nikki so well. According to Jerry:

"She really watches over the kids. She's a fabulous person, she's just unbelievable."

Nikki had general anesthesia each time she had proton treatments, due to her age. Because of Nikki's diagnosis, the craniotomy didn't remove all of her tumor, so proton beams targeted the remaining tumor. After proton treatments, aggressive chemo is applied to kill off any remaining cancer cells in her brain and other places that it might have spread to, like the spine.

At the Francis H. Burr Proton Therapy Center at MGH, Nikki had twenty proton treatments, ten on her spine and ten on her brain. She started treatments on April 20, 2015 and finished on May 17, 2015.

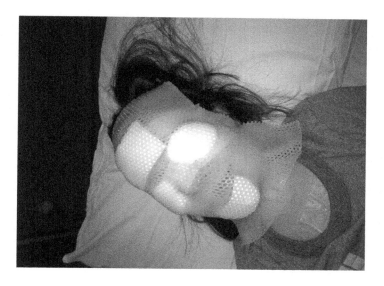

Nikki during proton treatments at MGH.

I asked Nikki how she felt during her proton treatments. She responded:

> *"It was awful. I could taste it. It was bad. I got so hot. It was so nerve-racking being the only one in the area because no one can come around you when you get radiation, so I listened to a Taylor Swift album. I could never listen to it again."*

As Nikki shared her story, I was overwhelmed by her strength, courage, grace, and calm. At fifty-two years old, I went through proton radiation. I remember what it was like being alone in the room with the sounds of the machine and the thoughts in my mind. I can't imagine being ten years old and going through it.

I asked Nikki if there was anything she could eat that comforted her during treatments. She said any kind of frappe, which is an ice-cream milk shake popular in the northeast. Pasta also helped.

If that's not tough enough, Nikki then underwent six months of grueling chemotherapy. Jerry said he'd never seen his daughter so sick. Maureen took Nikki to MGH on Mondays, and they would stay there for a week for her in-patient treatments.

Thankfully Nikki's proton treatments were approved by her insurance. Jerry had Blue Cross Blue Shield-A Plan. The insurance process was seemingly seamless for Nikki's parents.

Due to her diagnosis and side effects of cancer treatments, she lost all her hair and it's been difficult to grow back, so she sees a hair specialist and stays incredibly patient.

Nikki also doesn't produce enough hormones on her own. She checks in with her physician team at points throughout the year and she also sees an endocrinologist to treat her growth hormone. Nikki's growth hormone prescription costs $6,500 per month even with Jerry's current insurance plan, which is extremely frustrating for Jerry. He says:

"What the government doesn't see and what people don't understand is the cost of this disease is lifelong."

Nikki will be under medical care for the rest of her life. Every six months she has an MRI for surveillance. She recently had a brain bleed that was caught on the MRI, and since our interview, Nikki's had another round of scans and everything looked good!

Nikki just keeps on going. She's a superhero!

I asked Nikki if she had a mantra to stay strong. She responded:

"There is nothing to fear but fear itself."

Jerry taught Nikki this and it helped during many of the tough times.

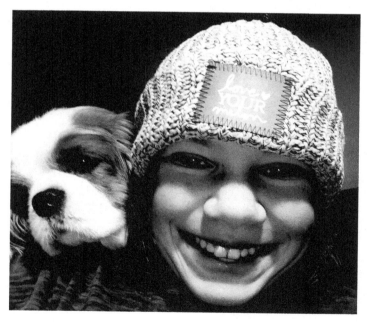

Nikki and her beloved dog JoJo.

Niki's dog, JoJo, an adorable Cavalier King Charles Spaniel, comforted Nikki throughout her diagnosis, treatment, and until this day. She sat at Nikki's feet while we chatted together over Zoom. Nikki also enjoyed the pet therapy dog Ed while she was in treatment at MGH.

Nikki, Maureen, and Jerry stay focused on the positives and are committed to giving back. In conjunction with MGH, after treatments ended Nikki raised funds for MGH's annual fundraiser for childhood cancer at the Boston Park Plaza Hotel. Still feeling extremely sick from treatments and weighing only fifty-eight pounds, Nikki received a standing ovation and walked the runway with her incredibly compassionate nurse, Rachel. Nikki was told her fundraising raised the most at the event.

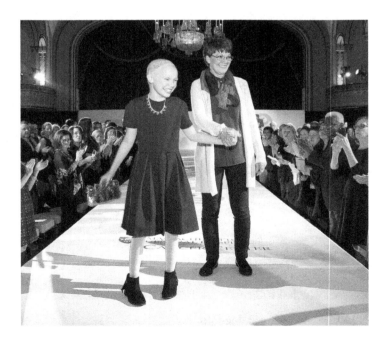

Nikki keeps going and gives back. Within three years, Nikki has raised over $30,000 which she has donated directly to MGH and the Children's Cancer Research. She's also closely involved with The Magical Moon Farm and Foundation in Marshfield, Massachusetts and The Wicked Good Cause located in Duxbury, Massachusetts. The month of September is dedicated to pediatric cancer. In recognition of this month, Nikki's designed her own t-shirt she sells to raise money for organizations.

Jerry gives back as well through MGH's Patient and Family Advisory Council (PFAC).

Nikki and her family can't say enough positive things about MGH's pediatric cancer unit located on the eighth floor at the hospital. Her medical team and nurses Rhonda and Rachel were phenomenal.

I can't say enough positive things about Nikki Schindler! Her strength, courage, and peaceful ways will make her the most successful child life specialist, which is Nikki's dream job once she graduates from college. Now a rising senior in the fall of 2021, there's no doubt in my mind that Nikki is Boston Strong and then some. If you're lucky to know Nikki, she will make you feel at ease. I would have never known all she's been through. Those of us who know Nikki are so lucky to have met her and learn from her.

For pediatric brain cancer patients and their families, we hope telling Nikki's story helps in understanding the medical process patients endure, while at the same time providing hope and strength. There truly is nothing to fear but fear itself. Nikki's taught us all that ultimate lesson.

PROTONS & PEDIATRIC CANCER

GRACE'S STORY

"Not everyone gets to attend the State of the Union address, and for the President to talk about me, that's pretty cool."

—GRACE ELINE, CANCER SURVIVOR, FOX NEWS

The American Childhood Cancer Organization featured Grace's heroic story with pediatric brain cancer as part of their Gold Ribbon Hero Award program. At four years old Grace Eline of Gillette, New Jersey was raising money for St. Jude Children's Research Hospital. In lieu of birthday gifts, she asked for donations. No one ever thought she would one day be in the fight herself.

Five years later she was rallying the neighborhood, friends, and family to raise money for childhood cancer during her own fight with brain cancer. She raised $40,000. By ten years old, she was sitting next to First Lady Melania Trump as President Trump's guest advocating for pediatric cancer at the nation's State of the Union Address.

I was introduced to Grace and her mom Aubrey through Jennifer Maggiore, the Executive Director of the National Association for Proton Therapy. Jennifer told me, if you are writing about pediatric cancer and protons you need to meet Grace and her mom Aubrey. She said Grace is so well respected and known for her passion to advocate, legislate, and help others, so off I went to hopefully meet Grace and Aubrey and learn about Grace's diagnosis, story, and journey with proton therapy.

In January of 2021, on a cold Friday afternoon, I met with Grace and Aubrey over Zoom. The minute the video turned on, there was Grace, smiling and ready to chat. Her warmth and sincerity would make anyone feel at home.

I asked Grace and Aubrey how they discovered Grace's cancer. In Aubrey's words, "Grace had symptoms for about two years—the most severe was extreme thirst and her growth significantly slowed down. Grace's pediatrician ran blood tests for two years, but nothing caused concern. Yet her growth continued to slow down."

"She was always off the charts for height until she wasn't."

After the second year of slowed growth, Grace was referred by her pediatrician to endocrinologist Ellen Oppenheimer, MD, RWJBarnabas Health. Dr. Oppenheimer ran a slew of tests and still nothing significant presented, so she was sent for an MRI. From this test, the initial tumor was detected on April 9, 2018. More tests came thereafter.

Through every blood draw, lumbar puncture, and long times spent getting scans like an MRI, bone scan, and PET scan,

Grace was emotionally strong and always positive. Her mom Aubrey described Grace's strength:

> *"She rose to the occasion through all of it without complaint, always wanting to help others."*

At nine years old on May 2, 2018, Grace was diagnosed with Germinoma—a germ cell brain tumor. According to St. Jude's Hospital, and the American Brain Tumor Association, this is a rare form of cancer in less than five percent of all brain tumors in children. Her aggressive cancer treatments began on May 7, 2018.

Suddenly Grace needed to trade her softball glove and gymnastics leotard for treatment gowns and even a Wonder Woman face mask she used to keep still during proton radiation treatments.

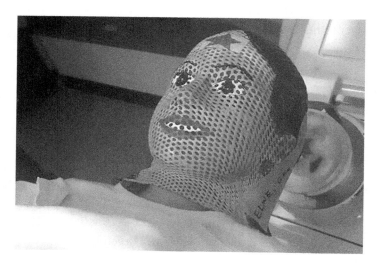

Grace, in her Wonder Woman mask during proton treatments.

On May 7, 2018, Grace began three days of chemotherapy, every three weeks, for four months at Newark Beth Israel Medical Center in Newark, New Jersey. Chemotherapy was rough on Grace. She vomited, lost her appetite at times, but powered through, never a complaint.

After her chemotherapy sessions were done, Grace started proton radiation treatments.

Because of the location of Grace's tumor, her neuro-oncologist Harini Rao, MD, Newark Beth Israel Medical Center, The Valerie Fund, prescribed proton radiation. **Photon radiation wasn't even in the conversation.**

According to the American Brain Tumor Association, "tumors are highly variable in their treatment and diagnosis." Some brain tumors are benign and treated conservatively and others are malignant and may require surgery, chemotherapy, and radiation. The goal of radiation therapy is to:

> *"Destroy tumor cells and prevent regrowth, while protecting the healthy tissue that surrounds the tumor. Proton therapy is typically recommended for the treatment of tumors that are irregularly shaped, located in hard-to-reach areas and/ or located near critical organs and brain tissue."*

With Dr. Rao's recommendation she met with Rahul Parikh, MD, Radiation Oncologist at Rutgers Cancer Institute of New Jersey. Dr. Parikh is also the Medical Director of the Laurie Proton Therapy Center at Robert Wood Johnson University Hospital.

The Elines also sought second and third opinions in New York City but returned to the teams in Newark and New Brunswick. The Elines felt Grace was in the best care possible, confident in the medical team and their expertise.

In RWJBarnabas Health Rutgers Cancer Institute of New Jersey, Let's Beat Cancer Together "Saving Grace," story, Dr. Parikh explained the case for proton:

> *"We have compelling data for patients of Grace's age and with her tumor location, it is standard of care to give her proton therapy. In the past, standard radiation to the brain would certainly cure a patient's tumor but likely result in real neuro-cognitive deficits.*

"For decades, the question was always: How do we treat this part of the brain, the suprasellar region, safely? Now, the modern treatment is chemotherapy followed by proton radiation and this has led to the highest cure rate and the lowest chance of secondary effects. I expect Grace to have a long-term cure because of how she was treated and how her tumor responded to all of her treatments. She should also continue to do extremely well in school."

In September through October 2018, Grace was treated at The Laurie Proton Therapy Center at Robert Wood Johnson University Hospital, in partnership with the Rutgers Cancer Institute of New Jersey. Grace received twenty-four rounds of proton radiation. That's a lot to go through at nine years old.

Through our talk, I asked Grace what she would tell a nine-year-old facing a brain cancer diagnosis, chemotherapy, and proton radiation. Grace said getting protons at the end of her treatment was like being at "the finish line." She said it's one step forward to getting to the end of treatment and she wants other pediatric patients to:

> *"Just relax and know you're in good hands. And just stay positive, smile, take it one day at a time. It'll get much better."*

Grace said that compared to chemo, proton radiation was a lot less stressful. She said she felt better, still had headaches, and was worn out at times, but at least she wasn't throwing up. That wasn't fun. She said it was also exciting because by the time she got to radiation, her hair started growing back.

When I went through treatments for breast cancer, I also stayed positive, but it was stressful. I wanted to know if Grace felt the same. She said:

> *"It was very stressful because I've never gotten bloodwork before, let alone been in an MRI machine for multiple hours at a time. It all happened so fast. So, the positioning that my tumor was in we didn't want to take any chances. So that was scary because it all happened in a blur. I don't remember a lot of it now because it happened so quickly, and I wasn't feeling good. It was a little bit scary, and it was kind of painful. But sometimes, I was quite happy when I got to go home. The staff were amazing there. They were very nice."*

Through it all, Grace carried her kindness and calmness during her experience with brain cancer. During treatment, she always smiled to help lighten the mood for the other patients she met along the way. Grace said having brain cancer isn't the most fun thing to go through, but she wouldn't trade the people she met and the friends she made for anything. I felt the same way when I finished treatments.

For all who know Grace, they describe her as very special. She's got a kind heart, infectious and beautiful smile. When Grace enters the room, she lightens the mood and fills those around her with positivity. I felt a sense of happiness chatting with Grace with her warm smile and kind ways. She's so poised, well-spoken, and she makes you feel so comfortable you forget she's twelve years old.

We chatted about Grace's journey with insurance approvals for proton radiation. Aubrey said she didn't have challenges with insurance approvals for proton radiation, not that she knew of. She said she heard from a lot of people it had been an issue for patients to get proton approved. In their case, it was okay. She said she never heard of a challenge with the insurance unless it happened behind the scenes. She's heard stories of other people being denied proton radiation and said it was heartbreaking to hear.

Based on the history of insurance denials, I asked Grace what she would like to say to legislators, not knowing at the time Grace was already very active advocating for pediatric cancer patients. Grace didn't hesitate. She said she thinks proton radiation is an important cause and maybe doesn't get the recognition it needs. She felt it's more common to see in pediatric brain cancers than maybe legislators even know. She said bringing "awareness and funding" is important, and boy, has Grace done her part and then some!

During treatments Grace was touched by The Valerie Fund. She told me:

"They took my mind away from what was going on at the moment, so when I was sad, they helped me by making me happy."

According to The Valerie Fund website, they are a charity in Maplewood, New Jersey, which was started when Ed and Sue Goldstein's daughter Valerie lost her life to cancer at nine years old.

Through Grace and Aubrey's journey with brain cancer, Aubrey said, "Our family expanded from our community that made cards and meal coordination to the hospitals at Rutgers Cancer Institute and the Valerie Fund at Newark Beth Israel."

About halfway through treatment, Aubrey found The Jay Fund who introduced her to a peer to peer support group, Momcology.org. According to Aubrey:

"That was the first time I really connected with other cancer moms. It was great. I was also raised to say positive and face any challenge with a fight and a good attitude. There was no other option, one day and one [step] at time. "

Along with her strength and positivity, Grace channeled her energy into helping others and in 2020, she founded her own initiative called the WITH Grace Initiative because paying it forward all started **with** Grace.

According to their website, WITH Grace supports pediatric cancer research initiatives and provides supplies and gifts of comfort to less fortunate families battling cancer, so each family can focus on their own fight with cancer. In 2020, through donations and fundraising efforts with local businesses, WITH Grace secured $46,376 in funding. According to the 2020 WITH Grace Initiative annual report, Grace's impact from these funds includes delivering care packages to seven hospitals in three states as well as helping local families, including purchasing crutches for cancer patients in need. They also started a kids committee which meets bi-weekly to brainstorm ways to help families and organizations in need.

Grace and her initiative actively advocate for pediatric funding to help end childhood cancer. Grace's mission is rooted in "acts of kindness toward others WITH Grace."

Grace is involved with childhood cancer in other ways.

On September 20, 2019, Grace was asked to speak as the pediatric cancer advocate at The Childhood Cancer Caucus. This annual bipartisan summit is a forum for members of Congress to work together to address pediatric cancer. The goal of the event is to raise awareness, advocate to prevent the pain, suffering, and long-term effects of childhood cancer, and ultimately work toward eradicating pediatric cancers.

As an advocate with The American Childhood Cancer Org (ACCO), Grace also spent time at Capitol Hill and The White House along with local lawmakers in New Jersey. Grace is so passionate and will do whatever she can to help people understand this disease is not easy and kids like her are in the fight and need help.

When I asked Aubrey how specifically Grace advocates, she answered:

"She advocates for more awareness and for the support and passing of Bills like the STAR Act, Gabriella Miller Kids First 2.0, Creating Hope Act, and CCDI Childhood Cancer Data Initiative. She was a voice at the then-VP Pence round table on pediatric cancer and is still called to round tables for these causes."

And her advocacy work is paying off!

Grace is currently working on three bills with New Jersey legislators.

On May 25, 2021, Grace and Aubrey joined Congressman Josh Gottheimer of New Jersey and northern Jersey medical experts, families, and cancer survivors to announce bipartisan legislation for federal investment in pediatric cancer research. Grace's advocacy was the headline on the Congressman's website! According to Congress.gov, on March 26, 2021, the **Fairness to Kids with Cancer Act of 2021** was introduced. The bill requires:

"The share of federal funds for cancer research that is allocated to pediatric cancer research to equal the percentage of the United States population that is under the age of 18."

How exciting! Grace is so driven, when I asked her where she saw her future in college and thereafter, she said:

> *"I want to be a pediatric neuro-oncologist. When I tell people, they're like: Can you say that in English for me? I tell them I want to be a children's cancer, brain, and spine doctor. There's so many different types of doctors and I was really impacted by all my doctors. I think I'd be a good doctor, and no offense to any of my doctors, I love them so much, but when they told me that something's not going to hurt, sometimes it feels the complete opposite way."*

Aubrey wants other parents and caregivers to know so many people are there to support pediatric patients. She said:

> *"Facing pediatric cancer is one of the scariest things you will ever have to encounter. There are people out there, strangers you've never even met, organizations and other patients, who want to help."*

While Grace will spend the rest of her life being monitored for recurrence of cancer, she currently shows no evidence of disease (NED), and is passionate about being the voice for kids with cancer and wants to help find a cure. She recovered well from proton radiation and is a positive voice for so many. She even shared her own story at the Alliance for Proton Therapy Access and was most recently one of two keynote speakers for the 2021 National Association for Proton Therapy's annual conference.

Although Grace planned on being in a clinical trial for proton radiation, her tissues were lost at the lab, not once, but twice.

Rather than dwelling on this misfortune, to help others, Aubrey now serves on the Patient Family Advisory Council (PFAC) at Newark Beth Israel Medical Center. In the research space for pediatric brain cancer both in the United States and worldwide, there are currently twelve studies listed on the clinicaltrials.gov website.

There's a lot of lessons to learned from Grace Eline. She takes things one day at a time with a smile and kindness. I was in awe of Grace when I interviewed her, and Aubrey, too. Grace's presence lights up the room. Her drive to help others navigate pediatric cancer, which many times includes a prescription for proton, is impressive.

I have no doubt in my mind the Eline family, with Grace's passion to help others, will be in the news for many years to come.

PROTONS & LYMPHOMA

———

KEELIN'S STORY

———

"I started chemotherapy and was told I might need radiation, so I saw a radiation oncologist and she recommended photon therapy, not protons. Then I asked about proton therapy, and suddenly it was the best idea ever."

—KEELIN MCGEE, CANCER SURVIVOR

Keelin and I met in 2019 through the Alliance for Proton Therapy Access, where Keelin had already been a volunteer for a year. I've always admired her calm and caring ways each time we interacted during our meeting with the Alliance.

Here's Keelin's story.

At twenty-seven years old, living in the Washington, DC area, Keelin worked as a government affairs coordinator at an oncology technology manufacturer. She had been offered the position there very soon after starting another job, so she almost turned it down.

Fate was on her side.

In 2017, Keelin went to her primary care doctor (PCP) on two separate occasions for a dry and persistent cough. She felt really rundown, and she just couldn't explain it. She told me:

> *"Both times my doctor kind of dismissed it thinking it was just a cold. I was told I would be fine."*

The second time she went to her PCP, she remembered being rushed. So, when her symptoms persisted, she didn't want to go back—she felt like a "nuisance."

Then she started developing severe chest pain. Each time she breathed in deeply, her chest radiated, and it kept getting worse. But she still felt couldn't go to her PCP. She thought: Maybe it would pass? But deep down she knew something was wrong.

Then she felt a little lump on her clavicle. She could move it around.

Within two weeks, it grew to the size of a golf ball.

So, she called her dad, who's a radiation oncologist, and he told Keelin to go to urgent care immediately. At urgent care, the doctor thought it might be an infected lymph node and referred her to an ear, nose, and throat (ENT) doctor.

She scheduled an appointment with the ENT and asked if she could be seen the next day. The ENT's receptionist fit her in the next day, saying it was an emergency which was a surprise to Keelin. In the meantime, Keelin started to worry:

"I knew something was wrong. I started Googling which is the last thing you should do—everything was leading to lymphoma."

So Keelin prepared herself for the worst.

Keelin was diagnosed with Stage IIA Hodgkin's lymphoma, and during this incredibly stressful time, she started a blog, which described:

> *"Following my CT scan, my Mom and I walked a CD with a copy of the results to send to my Dad to the FedEx store just down the street from my apartment. My heart had not stopped racing since we left the hospital, and my mind was completely scattered. As we were just about to send the CD off, my phone buzzed with a local number. My stomach immediately dropped, and my head started spinning. I answered, and just as I had suspected, it was my ENT doctor.*

> *"He sighed heavily, and I braced myself for the worst as tears poured out of my eyes. He asked where I was and told me to head to the emergency room as soon as possible. I lost all feeling in my body in a millisecond. He followed up by infamously telling me the lump in my neck was 'just the tip of the iceberg,' as I had fluid around my heart and there was a tumor in my chest pressing on the main vessel from my head to my heart—all signs pointing toward lymphoma. Without the decency to have me come in and tell me in person, the doctor left me to take the news like a bullet to the chest in the middle of a FedEx store. The emotional pain I felt in that instant far surpassed any other*

pain I had ever felt. I was completely shattered and made to feel as though I was dying. There was no reassurance and I thought, this was it.

"By the grace of God, I had my mom with me, and we spilled into the street outside, hailing a cab instantly. On the way to the ER, I called my boyfriend, Neil, to let him know the news. For all his questions, I did not have any answers and imagined how helpless he was feeling on the other side of the world. The timing could not have been worse as he had just left the night before to go home to Ireland for two weeks.

"Within five minutes, we were at the ER and I was made to think by the doctor that someone was going to be waiting for me and would come down to see me. However, when we arrived, we were told I would just have to wait my turn for a bed as they were full, and the doctor never came to check on me. Instead, my mom and I had to sit in the waiting room sobbing as I kept asking her if I was going to die."

According to Cancer.net, in 2020 an estimated 8,480 of Hodgkin lymphoma cases will be diagnosed, which represents .00047 percent of estimated cancer diagnoses in 2020.

Like other cancers, Hodgkin's lymphoma also has different stages. The cancer staging system like Stage I or II is used to describe how much the cancer has spread. The letter behind the number in Hodgkin's lymphoma indicates:

- Loss of more than ten percent of body weight over the previous six months (without dieting)

- Unexplained fever of at least 100.4°F (38°C)
- Drenching night sweats

According to the American Cancer Society, patients with these symptoms are categorized with the B behind the stage number like IIB. B type is more advanced which requires a more aggressive treatment. Keelin was diagnosed with IIA which meant she didn't present with these symptoms of the B type. Yet being diagnosed with any stage of cancer is equally as scary.

Keelin's symptoms included pain in her chest which affected her breathing and almost sent her into heart failure. She was extremely fatigued and had a persistent cough. She also had the lump in her neck that grew.

Her experience at the hospital was so stressful, almost no words can describe it. Because of this, she was transferred to Johns Hopkins Medicine in Baltimore, Maryland, where she remained for about a week. Her oncologist Richard F Ambinder, MD, PhD, Director of the Division of Hematologic Malignancies, Professor of Oncology, ran other tests, including a PET scan which doctors use to detect cancer metastases in the body.

After the tests, she started chemotherapy at the hospital. She continued eight chemo treatments throughout the following months. While at the hospital, she reflected on her recent one-year anniversary in her current role at the oncology technology manufacturer:

> *"If I had worked anywhere else, I would have had great difficulty. Given the work of my company in oncology,*

everyone was incredibly understanding when I took days off for chemotherapy and worked from home."

After four chemo treatments, Keelin had another PET scan to see how she was responding to treatment. The scan still showed a sizeable tumor in her chest, and Dr. Ambinder sent her to a radiation oncologist for a consultation.

During this appointment, she was prescribed photon radiation as the next step in her cancer treatment after finishing all eight rounds of chemo. Keelin's dad and sister are both radiation oncologists and encouraged Keelin to ask the doctor about proton therapy. Because of her work, Keelin was also aware of the benefits of proton therapy.

When Keelin asked about protons, it suddenly became "the best idea ever" to receive proton treatment. This is frustrating to me as Keelin isn't the first patient to tell me they weren't originally prescribed proton radiation because the physician either didn't offer it at their cancer center or maybe weren't familiar with its benefits.

Her doctor was supportive of the idea and recommended treatment at a few proton centers, including Cincinnati Children's Hospital.

Keelin selected John C. Breneman, MD, Medical Director, Cincinnati Children's Hospital Medical Center, UC Health Proton Therapy Center, for her treatment. She moved to Cincinnati to receive treatment, with the support of her employer. Cincinnati Children's is one of only two proton centers in the world owned by a children's hospital. It's located on Cincinnati Children's campus.

As happens to so many patients, the insurance process began, and the stress mounted.

Dr. Breneman submitted her case for prior authorization and approval for proton radiation. While Keelin waited for the approval she thought:

> *"Through my role at work, I was knowledgeable on legislation and reimbursement related to radiotherapy, understanding the challenges in accessing proton therapy for cancer patients who had been prescribed this treatment. What I didn't know was that I was soon going to be one of those patients."*

Keelin had Anthem insurance, and they denied approval for proton treatment on the first try.

Dr. Breneman appealed her case and had a peer-to-peer review with another physician at the insurance company who reviewed Keelin's case.

Her treatment was denied a second time:

> *"My denial came during the worst week of my recovery from chemo. I was severely neutropenic (low white blood cell count) and anemic (low red cell count), and it was difficult to leave my bed, let alone try to fight my insurer.*
>
> *"I laid in bed thinking how unfair it was for someone who did not know my case well, to deny me access to treatment*

that would help save my life. How dare they defy the advice of an expert prescribing this treatment?"

As fate would have it, Keelin's move into her role at the oncology manufacturer, a self-funded insurance company, provided options for Keelin. She recalled:

"I worked through the appeal process with the Human Resources manager at my work. My case was ultimately raised to our CEO who got involved and agreed to cover the cost of my cancer treatment."

Before Keelin's CEO got involved, her family had started making plans on how to pay out of pocket for treatments. They considered taking out loans and other ways to pay.

Yet the CEO's decision was a huge relief for Keelin. She already knew so much about proton radiation versus photon for her case. She wasn't going back to photon treatment. Again, her sister and dad, both radiation oncologists, were firm in their belief Keelin should have proton treatments.

On September 14, 2017, Keelin started proton treatments.

Keelin received seventeen rounds of proton treatments and her side effects were fatigue, sunburn-like redness on her chest, and pain swallowing. "All a walk in the park compared to chemo," Keelin said.

Here's Keelin's advice for patients navigating their cancer diagnosis:

"Trust your gut. It sounds like the biggest cliché, but I think a lot of people didn't believe me. They didn't believe me that I had cancer because I was so young. No matter your age, you can advocate for yourself throughout your cancer journey. I wanted to know every single option I could. It mattered to me."

If Keelin had gone with the original recommended treatment from her doctor, she would have had photon radiation, but she wasn't going to accept that opinion. That's hard for patients to do.

Even outside of radiation, my plastic surgeon Ariel Rad, MD, PhD, Sherber + Rad Washington, DC, was so patient with me. When I asked him what kind of surgery I should have after reviewing the options he presented, he thoroughly reviewed the pros and cons of each. He spent an hour with my husband and me. His expertise, calm yet confident ways, and his ability to communicate in laymen's terms with such sincere compassion made all the difference for me. He also made me feel comfortable when I told him I already had another appointment with a different plastic surgeon I had already booked before we met.

I reached out to Dr. Rad when publishing this book. He's an incredible physician and I wanted to know his thoughts about patients empowering themselves. Dr. Rad said:

"I encourage patients to seek other opinions to determine what's right for them to have the safest outcome, while minimizing downtime and maximizing results."

I couldn't agree more. When I saw the other plastic surgeon, within five minutes of my exam, my husband looked at me and smiled. We already knew Dr. Rad was the surgeon for me.

As Keelin mentioned, patients should seek all options and feel good about doing so. It's all about advocacy and speaking up. She also said:

> *"I think of other young adults, and if they don't ask those questions, radiation can have a huge impact on a patient's heart, lungs, reproductive organs. In my case, my heart and lungs would have been significantly affected by photon treatment."*

As for insurance, Keelin recommends working on this process with a friend, family member, or someone at work who can help navigate this difficult process in healthcare.

I agree, it's so difficult figuring out insurance alone, especially after cancer treatments or surgery. Patients are scared and tired and just want to get into treatment and get rid of the cancer. So, it's important to let go sometimes and let others help.

> *"Surrendering parts of the insurance process can be difficult to handle, but it's worth it to preserve a patient's energy and time,"* said Keelin.

Four years later, Keelin is doing great. She has moved into a new department within the same company, working to improve cancer care for patients just like herself around the world.

She also graduated in May of 2021 with her Master's Degree in Global Health Planning and Management from Johns Hopkins University. She authored her Capstone paper at Hopkins on improving access to mental health services for rural cancer patients.

Both of us have our own fears and worries around cancer recurrence. We are blessed protons helped save our lives and minimized dreadful side effects that could have had life altering consequences, but cancer recurrence is a topic we both deal with.

During our interview, Keelin and I talked about the fear of cancer recurrence in that sometimes survivors don't ever really stop thinking about it. It's different for everyone, but most of us feel at some point we are looking over our shoulder, worrying it might come back. My college roommate Annie felt the same. She was diagnosed four years before me and said right after treatments ended her fear was greater than it is was for every year thereafter. Fear of recurrence for Annie got better with time.

In Living Well Beyond Cancer, Conversations on Survivorship at the Dana-Farber Institute, Amy Gross, MSW, LICSW discussed, "fear of cancer recurrence is the most central thing cancer survivors talk about when they come for counselling."

Somehow this is comforting to me. Amy talked about a patient who described the fear of cancer like a house. Right after treatment, her mind was like a house, each room represented cancer coming back. Overtime, the fear is like having a backroom. It's there, but day to day, you don't spend time in that room. I like that analogy.

As Keelin said to me, "I know the cancer is gone, but any slight cough felt like it could be cancer to me."

Keelin's commitment to contributing to the topic of fear of recurrence through her Capstone at school was her way of paying it forward.

Keelin is full of gratefulness. Apart from her incredible medical team, she has immense gratitude for her mom and now-husband, Neil. As her primary caregivers, Keelin said she would have been lost without them.

She's also grateful for her dad and sister, Mackenzie, for helping her through all the stressful phone calls and questions regarding her diagnosis and treatment options.

Her siblings, Colin and Caitlin, their spouses, and all her nieces and nephews helped in their support and love during her diagnosis, treatment, and thereafter.

Her family, friends, and coworkers also kept her going and supported through treatment and survivorship when it felt impossible. She concluded:

> "Most importantly, in honor of my Aunt Maureen, [who is] the reason I will never stop advocating for cancer patients and survivors."

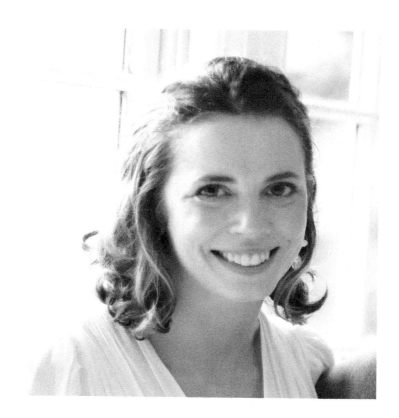

Keelin's wedding day.

PROTONS & THYMUS CANCER

EVA'S STORY

"On September 8, 2016, I had a CT scan of my chest wall. Before I even got to the first traffic light from the imaging center, I received a call from the doctor. He asked me if I was in a place where I could talk. I told him no, I'm in my car, but I'm fine and I'm calm."

—EVA TAI, CANCER SURVIVOR

At fifty-one years old, Eva Tai, an industrial engineer living in Charlotte, North Carolina with her husband and daughter, had just returned from a cruise. She suddenly felt an unusual type of fatigue and spasm on her left chest. Eva had a history of celiac disease and fibromyalgia, so she was used to symptoms of fatigue, but this was different, so she called her primary care doctor to check it out.

Her doctor was on vacation, so Eva was seen by another physician. Since she had chest pain, the doctor gave her a prescription for chest spasms and sent her for tests. After the CT test and at the traffic light, Eva learned she had a thymoma, which is a tumor on the thymus which may or may not have been cancerous.

The thymus is a gland located in the chest wall between the lungs and behind the breastbone. It is located just in front of and above the heart. It's part of the lymphatic and immune systems, so its function is vital in fighting new illnesses from bacterial and fungal infections.

The America Cancer Society defines thymoma cancer as cancer cells that form on the outside surface of the thymus. Treatment involves surgery, chemotherapy, or radiation, sometimes all three depending on the diagnosis. Less than one percent out of 1.5 million people develop thymoma. This means about four hundred people per year develop the disease.

Back at the traffic light, Eva listened and then told the doctor she knew all about thymoma. Her sister had thymoma cancer ten years ago. Eva's doctor said she needed a biopsy as the next step toward diagnosis.

Eva started to do additional research and used alternative medicine treatments in hopes to shrink the tumor. She wanted to talk to her primary care doctor for clarification on her next steps. Once back from vacation, her primary doctor explained although it's most common for the tumor to be a thymoma, there was a small chance it could be a lymphoma, which would be treated by an oncologist without surgery. She agreed Eva's next steps would be to get the tumor biopsied.

On October 17, 2015, as the imaging staff took another scan of the tumor and prepared her for the biopsy, Eva found out her tumor was significantly reduced by 70 percent. As a result, she decided to continue with alternative medicine treatments and monitor the tumor.

For three years, the tumor decreased in size on every scan until August 2019. The size went up slightly, so the plan was to have another scan in three months.

But, Eva had already planned a big family vacation to Asia in December. She decided to go on vacation and deal with her biopsy when she got back. All the doctors agreed it wouldn't be a problem to wait until the New Year.

She came back to the United States on New Year's Eve from Hong Kong just as the novel coronavirus disease started to simmer in China. Eva was well prepared on her trip. She wore a mask the entire time of her trip and maintained her social distance when she interacted with others.

When she got back, she completed her biopsy and her surgeon diagnosed Eva with type IIB Thymoma. At that time, she was given all the details of a minimally invasive robotic thymectomy as her next step.

On February 4, 2020, Eva had surgery to remove the thymoma. Her husband was expecting a two-hour surgery. Instead, the surgery took roughly seven hours. By the time he saw her, it was around 7:00 p.m. in the intensive care unit. He told her she had had an open chest surgery because they found carcinogen cells from the robotic procedure.

The next day, she recalled, the surgeon told her there were carcinogen cells, and the tumor was removed close to her heart, so part of the pericardium was removed. From Medline Plus's article "Pericardial Disorders," the pericardium is a membrane, or sac, that surrounds the heart. It holds the heart in place and helps it work properly.

Cancer wasn't on the top of Eva's mind during her two-night stay at the hospital. She was busy with breathing exercises, tube removal, pain management, and working on the ability to eat and sleep and walk. She was able to start walking the next day following her stay in the ICU.

On Feb 21, 2020, Eva had her follow up appointment with her surgeon. At this point, everyone was wearing a face mask and her husband couldn't accompany her in the room. Eva asked more specific questions:

> *"Isn't thymoma IIB not cancerous with no carcinogenic cells? Do I have cancer? Do I need radiation?"*

She left the appointment a bit confused with the conversation, but her surgeon told her to meet with a radiation oncologist as her next step, so she booked an appointment.

On March 2, 2020, Eva met with Matthew Ward, MD, Radiation Oncologist, Atrium Health Levine Cancer Institute—Morehead. At this appointment, she discussed her concerns about radiation and why she favored against it. She was supposed to start radiation within three months of surgery.

But Dr. Ward recommended proton radiation. Because of the location of the tumor and the fact protons would more effectively protect her heart, tissues, and other structures, he recommended Eva to the Maryland Proton Treatment Center (MPTC) located in Baltimore, Maryland. Like many of us who have had proton treatment, Eva hadn't heard of it either. After hearing the doctor describe the benefits of a more targeted therapy, radiation sounded promising.

Eva had friends in the DC area, having previously lived in Silver Spring, Maryland, so she was familiar with the area. She thought relocating to Maryland with her husband for about a month was doable.

Eva started to research protons. She reviewed MedStar Georgetown University Hospital Proton Therapy Center in Washington, DC, which opened in March of 2018. She also found Emory Proton Center in Atlanta, Georgia, which opened in December 2018.

She also researched MPTC. It opened in June of 2016 and was the most established and the largest proton center compared to the others. MPTC also offered help with lodging, which is something Eva needed as she would relocate there from North Carolina for a month to undergo twenty-eight days of treatment.

Eva felt confident about her decision to be treated there. Her doctor, Robert Miller, MD, Radiation Oncologist, had experience treating thymomas which is sometimes hard to find. Having a doctor with this clinical specialty eased Eva's worries.

On March 6, 2020, Eva started the new patient inquiry process at MPTC.

On March 11, 2020, the World Health Organization (WHO) declared the novel coronavirus disease a global pandemic.

On March 13, the Center for Disease Control (CDC) in the United States declared a national emergency concerning the COVID-19 outbreak.

By March 17, 2020, COVID-19 cases had escalated in the United States. Many states went on lockdown, preventing people from leaving their homes except for essential trips like medical appointments and grocery store visits. This lockdown was intended to prevent the spread of infection and not overwhelm hospitals with cases. Healthcare providers were treating COVID-19 patients and cancelling medical appointments, and telemedicine was created seemingly overnight.

As such, Eva's first appointment scheduled with Dr. Miller on March 30, 2020, was postponed. Eventually she was seen for a telemedicine appointment on April 20, 2020.

Eva's initial prior authorization on April 29, 2020, was sent to Anthem Blue Cross Blue Shield PPO. Her insurance plan was self-insured through her husband Chester's employer. Allison Scull, Referral Coordinator, Manager for MPTC, and Dr. Miller handled her case.

Due to the global pandemic and insurance delays, on May 26, 2020, Eva had her first in-person appointment with Dr. Miller, roughly fifteen weeks after surgery in February.

Because her insurance was already declined twice, Dr. Miller assembled a comparative plan, which meant he put together more information comparing traditional photon versus proton radiation and why this was a superior treatment for Eva's case.

Before treatment started, Eva and Chester decided to pay out of pocket with a credit card for the total amount of treatment, which was $42,000.

Eva started treatment on June 15, 2020.

On June 16, 2020 Eva's case was overturned.

Eva confirmed her timeline with Allison Scull at the proton center:

1. 4/29/2020—prior authorization submitted to insurance.
2. 5/1/2020—case number assigned and acknowledged by insurance.
3. 5/4/2020—proton treatment denied (was advised by case nurse, a peer to peer review didn't have the option to overturn the case and an appeal would need to be submitted).
4. 5/5/2020—first level of appeal submitted to insurance with letter of medical necessity (LMN) completed by physician.
5. 5/6/2020—insurance confirmed receipt of appeal.
6. 5/12/2020—first level appeal denied.
7. 5/12/202—second level of appeal submitted.
8. 6/3/2020—comparative plan completed and submitted to insurance.
9. 6/9/2020—second level appeal denied.

10. 6/10/2020—external appeal submitted (including comparative plan).
11. 6/16/2020—external appeal overturned denial and approved.

By her second week of treatment, on June 26, 2020, Eva received a **refund check for the $42,000**. She felt so lucky and relieved.

When we spoke, I was so frustrated for Eva, Chester, Allison, and Dr. Miller who went through eleven steps to get Eva's insurance provider to pay for treatment. The prior authorization, peer to peer review denial, and appeal circle of failure is so unfair to patients.

The American Society for Radiation Oncology surveyed 620 radiation oncologists in 2019 regarding prior authorization, and 62 percent of the physicians said their cases were ultimately overturned.

Through the back and forth of the insurance process, Eva kept calm and focused on treatment, but as she told her story, I couldn't help but think how stressful it must have been, especially during a global pandemic.

While in treatment, Eva walked with her husband every day. The walks kept her upbeat and positive. She had minimal side effects from radiation. It wasn't until the last two weeks of treatment that Eva's skin was discolored.

Conversely, photon radiation, short-term side effects could have been worse:

- Skin irritation or changes where the radiation goes into your body. This can be like a bad sunburn. Your skin may blister and peel.
- Nausea
- Fatigue
- Irritation of the esophagus. This could lead to eating problems such as pain when swallowing.
- Loss of appetite and weight loss

According to Cedars Sinai, long-term side effects can be even more challenging such as:

- Lung damage from radiation which could lead to trouble breathing and shortness of breath.
- Increased risk of heart disease. This includes heart attacks.
- Secondary cancers, especially in the treatment area.

After surgery and throughout Eva's treatments, she stayed focused on others versus thinking about herself. Between March and May, Eva made over 250 medical masks for people to wear to protect themselves from the COVID-19 virus.

Almost a year after surgery, Eva's doing great! She's retired from Bank of America and enjoys her walks and time with her family. She's so appreciative of the team at MPTC, and so am I.

Eva is grateful for her daughter Carissa, who called her often from college to check on her progress. She's also grateful for her husband Chester, who supported her and told her not to worry about money. He drove her everywhere and helped her with all the billing and paperwork. He cooked for her and helped her to stay positive.

In hindsight, Eva thought her surgery recovery and the six-weeks of proton therapy would be the most challenging year of her life. She told me:

"It turned out the surgery recovery was seamless, and the six weeks of proton therapy were really the best time I had in that year. The side effects from proton were minimal, and I enjoyed a therapy vacation walking with different groups of friends in Maryland, Virginia, and Washington, DC."

If Eva had the chance to talk to legislators about the insurance prior authorization and peer review process, I asked her what she would like to say. She answered:

"Why do insurance companies need a third party to evaluate and judge and approve protons when there is already so much information out there, scientific information, proving the efficacy of proton radiation? Even as a patient, I'm able to Google proton and see the benefit. To me, it's so obvious, but I guess it isn't obvious to the insurance professionals?"

Why aren't our legislators involved in policies to fix this? After all, according to the NCBI, "the goal of health policy is to protect and promote the health of individuals and the community."

In "Which Industry Spends the Most on Lobbying?" by Jake Frankenfield, it turns out over the past twenty-two years, the pharmaceutical and health products industry has spent the most money of all industries in lobbying legislators second only to health insurance. As such, insurance companies have been heavily involved in lobbying looking to "influence new regulations."

It seems it's an uphill battle hearing the significant influence health insurance companies have with legislators through their lobbying efforts. For this reason, our patient stories like Eva's must be told.

Patients have reached out and asked me if I have heard of anyone paying for proton radiation and then getting their money back. Eva's story is one of hope, not only because she's doing so well after her cancer, but also because she paid out of pocket and got her money back.

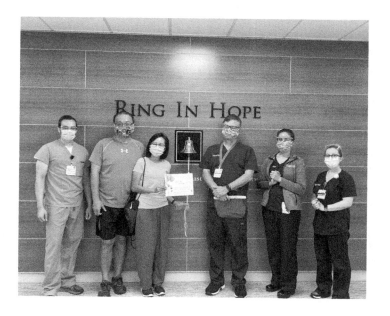

Eva ringing the Hope Bell.

ABOUT ADVOCACY

"I really love sharing my story and advocating for proton therapy. I spoke at the MD Anderson Proton Conference in 2015 and my doctor told me I was the only person he knew of who has ever received a standing ovation from the medical community. It was a humbling experience."

—CATHLEEN MCBURNEY, CANCER SURVIVOR

I met Cathleen through our volunteer work at the Alliance for Proton Therapy Access. You'll hear more of Cathleen's inspiring story of faith in the next chapter.

The words *advocacy* and *advocate* are used quite a bit in healthcare with different meanings, starting with patients finding their own voice through speaking up.

But how do patients speak up and advocate for themselves, with their own voice and opinion, about their own care?

It's tough. When I was diagnosed with breast cancer it was scary and things moved so fast. I wasn't the expert and relied on my medical staff to cure me. Yet by the time I learned about radiation, I started finding my own voice. By April of 2018, a month after surgery, I asked a ton of questions. I found my voice, and my medical team was so patient.

Sometimes patients are afraid to speak up, not wanting to offend or go against the doctor's orders. I found, through the patients I interviewed, most of us spoke up and asked if protons would be right for us. We advocated and decided with the doctor what the best treatment plan should be, only then to be faced with delays and insurance denials for treatment where a more persistent and determined voice was needed.

Through more than twenty-five interviews with patients, physicians, advocates, patient experience leaders, lawyers, and caregivers, I asked:

What should a patient know about advocacy?

"Dr. Casolaro, our team doctor, came along with me when we first met with Dr. Bajaj. Dr. Casolaro was an advocate for me and suggested proton therapy. After insurance denied my treatments, Dr. Bajaj called my insurance company on my behalf and told them this would be the best treatment for me along with the chemo plan they had, and it was agreed upon. And they agreed to do it, that same day."

—HEAD COACH RON RIVERA, WASHINGTON FOOTBALL TEAM

"I think patients have to be their own advocate. They have to get their provider to provide them with the knowledge and the bullet points and pieces of information about what to take to their insurance company to appeal their case for treatment."

—ARPIT CHHABRA, MD, RADIATION ONCOLOGIST, DIRECTOR
OF EDUCATION, NEW YORK PROTON CENTER

"Part of the willingness to advocate is to be an expert in your own condition, and it doesn't even have to be about your disease. I'm not saying patients are experts in their disease, a doctor clearly knows, clinically, the best path forward. But we can advocate for how we live in that space and how we engage with the realities of where we find ourselves."

—JASON WOLF, CEO, THE BERYL INSTITUTE

"No matter your age, you can advocate for yourself throughout your cancer journey. Patients should ask for every single treatment option available and then ask: 'What are the side effects, short and long term?' Based on the location of my tumor, photon radiation could have had a potentially large impact on my heart, lungs, and breast tissue. Working through insurance, patients should have a support system and rely on them because it's so hard do it alone. I surrendered that piece. I was just too tired from chemo to battle the insurance company. Ask the cancer center where you're being treated about what resources they have to help. With the insurance process, advocating for yourself and also relying on those around you to help is the best advice I can give."

—KEELIN MCGEE, CANCER SURVIVOR

"There's a lack of awareness about the role of proton therapy for cancer treatment in Canada. I feel it is important to increase awareness about protons as a treatment option. For example, we held a symposium in 2018 on proton therapy in Ontario to discuss how we can take this advanced cancer treatment forward in our province. We wanted to raise awareness amongst physicians and patients alike, because even amongst some of my Canadian colleagues, there's a prevailing perception that since we don't have easy access to protons, this treatment option can be out of sight and out of mind. I also wrote an op-ed piece in a national newspaper about how protons can be useful in many clinical situations, especially for children. I continue to try to raise awareness regarding this unmet health care need for cancer patients in our country."

—DEREK TSANG, MD, RADIATION ONCOLOGIST AT THE PRINCESS MARGARET CANCER CENTRE IN TORONTO, CANADA

"We've definitely learned we can all work together to advocate and raise awareness by making lots of noise. That's what cancer needs, especially childhood cancers."

—JERRY SCHINDLER, FATHER OF NIKKI SCHINDLER, CANCER SURVIVOR

"Advocate for yourself. There are a lot of organizations out there like the Alliance for Proton Therapy Access, connect with them. There are support groups that know what you're going through and can be there for you."

—MARIAM TARIQ, CANCER SURVIVOR

"Patients need to push back when doctors ignore their concerns. Even if you're younger, listen when your body is telling you something is off. I talked to experienced, intelligent medical staff that disagreed with my concerns, but I'm glad I kept pushing. I knew something wasn't right and when I finally got someone to listen my breast cancer had already spread."

—JILLIAN BENSTEIN, CANCER SURVIVOR

"Early in my career, I was fortunate to be an early promoter of proton therapy in the United States. Fifteen years later, I am still a passionate advocate for this powerful cancer therapy. I have always said **proton therapy is the only cancer treatment with a fan club,** *so I recently created the Proton Fight Club. This platform is a national social media advocacy program to help build awareness for one of the most advanced cancer treatments in the world."*

—BILL HANSEN, PRESIDENT OF BLUE ORCA MARKETING

"It's about asking, what is the best service we can provide to the residents of Northern Virginia? What is the legacy we leave behind in terms of cancer care for our patients, our families, and our friends who live here? And it wasn't until we started thinking about it in that context, as a collective group, that we should advocate to have this technology in Northern Virginia. And then we embarked upon this three-year process to make sure we did that, and we got it."

—GOPAL K. BAJAJ, MD, MBA RADIATION ONCOLOGIST, PRESIDENT, RADIATION ONCOLOGY ASSOCIATES, PC, VICE CHAIR OF THE GOVERNMENT RELATIONS COUNCIL FOR THE ASTRO BOARD OF DIRECTORS

Next, patient advocates are professionals who work on a patient's behalf to help navigate the healthcare system with the goal of gaining access to the system, helping patients through insurance, financial, and other healthcare needs.

Many of the proton treatment centers are used to patients being declined by insurance for proton treatment. The centers have a process in which patients can work with their own physician and a representative from the center who can help patients navigate insurance denials and appeals.

Dr. Eblan and Allison at MPTC encouraged me to speak up and call UnitedHealthcare and advocate for myself, which I did. But I wanted to do more when I was in the thick of insurance denials. I researched and couldn't find advocacy resources for breast cancer and proton radiation patients.

So, I thought sharing some resources for patients might be helpful as it's overwhelming finding advocacy groups when a patient's first been diagnosed.

There are different types of organizations that can help patients in different ways.

The Alliance for Proton Therapy Access is specific to proton radiation. When I became a part of this organization through volunteering as a proton champion, I learned so much about patient advocacy by first sharing my story. Molly Daniels, Executive Director, and her team of hard-working professionals are there to help patients share their stories, even some with the media, in hopes the insurance companies will overturn their cases. The Alliance is an excellent resource with one goal in mind: to help patients gain access to proton therapy by sharing their stories, sometimes with the media.

The Patient Advocate Foundation (PAF), a national 501(c)(3) nonprofit charity, works directly with patients with chronic, life threatening, and debilitating diseases access the healthcare system and follow through on the plan of care prescribed by the doctor. Their website is chock full of video testimonials and patient resources. The National Patient Advocate Foundation is a sister organization to the PAF which works on the policy level on behalf of patients.

There are different types of cancer related organizations that can also help such as American Cancer Society, breastcancer.org, Cure for Lymphoma Research Foundation, Patient Access Network Foundation, Side Effect Support, LLC, and more.

One of the most impressive and compassionate themes from all the physicians I interviewed is advocacy. Each physician I spoke to advocates for their patients. Day in and day out, they are working with patients to heal, cure, or manage a cancer diagnosis, yet they are also seemingly managing another day job, which is getting their patients access to treatment. Whether in the United States or in Dr. Tsang's case in Canada, each physician dedicates endless hours of paperwork fighting for access to cancer treatments for their patients. It's so disheartening to hear this extra workload placed on physicians. Not one physician complained about this process when we spoke. It's part of their role. Yet at the same time, I could hear their frustration.

I found my own voice through my fight with my insurance company and advocated for myself. I encourage patients to do the same. Ask about proton treatment. It's not the right treatment for every cancer diagnosis, but it might be the right one for you.

For a robust list of advocacy resources, visit the Association of Community Cancer centers https://www.accc-cancer.org/state-societies. who are "the leading education and advocacy organization for the cancer care community."

CATHLEEN'S STORY OF ADENOID CYSTIC CARCINOMA, ADVOCACY, & FAITH IN GOD

"My advocacy started when I said to myself, 'I no longer accept what you are telling me. I need to figure it out on my own.' Advocacy is about finding your voice."

—CATHLEEN MCBURNEY, CANCER SURVIVOR

For ten years Cathleen McBurney, an advocate and patient engagement manager, had severe jaw pain. She repeatedly visited her primary care doctor in California who told Cathleen her pain was temporomandibular disorder (TMJ). Over time, she started losing feeling on the right side of her face and was experiencing nerve pain. She thought maybe it was Bell's palsy, a condition which causes weakness in the muscles of the face. Instead, her primary care doctor diagnosed her with a pinched nerve. Cathleen carried on with the pain, trusting her plan of care and medical team.

In 2011, having lived in California for many years, Cathleen and her husband decided to move to Texas to be closer to family. The move and the days, weeks, and months thereafter were life-altering for Cathleen. It was a move that saved her life.

In April of 2013, after she celebrated her mother's seventieth birthday, she woke up from her sleep and felt like someone had a knife and stabbed her in the face.

> *"I'm not exaggerating. I felt like someone had a knife and was repeatedly stabbing me, and I was screaming in pain running around the house. I never even had headaches before, and I was running around the house trying to find something to help take away the pain. I now know the pain was the tumor invading my trigeminal nerve."*

The next day, Cathleen called her friend who was a retired neurologist for guidance. He found a local neurologist who quickly discovered upon examination that something was definitely wrong. He sent her for an MRI a few days later. Cathleen's mom accompanied her on the twenty-minute drive to the imaging location in Austin, Texas. After the MRI, they weren't even home for five minutes when she received the call from her neurologist saying:

"You have a tumor the size of a large plum completely filling your entire sinus cavity."

It was at this time Cathleen became her own advocate. Over the years, Cathleen had had multiple sinus infections, jaw pain, numbness, and now she understood why. The tumor was invading her sinus cavity. Not one doctor in California even suggested an MRI. This is when Cathleen found her voice.

Cathleen's advocacy started with her diagnosis. She now knew she would need to ask more questions she might not have before. She spoke up. She found her voice, and she encourages others to do the same.

After seeing an ear, nose, and throat (ENT) doctor, Peter Scholl DDS, MD, FACS, who biopsied the tumor, Cathleen was diagnosed with Stage IV inoperable adenoid cystic carcinoma (ACC), an extremely rare head and neck cancer that affects about 1,200 people a year in the United States according to Cancer.net. Cathleen told me:

> "When I got the call, it was cancer, I fell to the floor and sobbed. I immediately asked the Lord to take it from me. Not necessarily the cancer, but the burden of it."

She was sent to Ehab Y. Hanna, MD, FACS, an internationally recognized head and neck surgeon. Dr. Hanna is Professor and Vice Chair of the Department of Head and Neck Surgery at the University of Texas MD's Anderson Cancer Center in Houston, Texas.

Dr. Hanna recommended proton radiation for Cathleen's tumor and requested she see Steven J. Frank, MD, Professor of Radiation Oncology at the University of Texas's MD Anderson Cancer Center, and Medical Director of the Proton Therapy Center at MD Anderson. As head and neck cancers are his specialty and Dr. Frank had also treated another ACC patient with protons, Cathleen would benefit from his expertise and experience.

Within an hour, Cathleen was seen by Dr. Frank.

By this time she knew she had to have radiation to reduce the size of the tumor. Cathleen was forty-four at the time. She had never heard of proton radiation prior to her treatment.

Dr. Hanna explained having proton treatment was her only chance of living a life with or without cancer. After suffering in pain for ten years, and based on the size of the tumor, they hoped to treat Cathleen's condition more like a chronic disease whereby the radiation would improve her jaw mobility and pain by shrinking the tumor.

With ACC, there is no known cure. Prior to proton therapy, patients were often treated with debilitating surgeries and/or photon radiation, which had significant side effects for many patients. Because of Cathleen's diagnosis and because she was a healthy forty-four-year-old, this worked to her advantage to have proton radiation to treat her cancer.

Cathleen's medical team sent her insurance information in for prior authorization and Cathleen remembered getting a letter in the mail from her insurance that proton radiation wasn't covered for her treatment despite her doctor's recommendation. She said:

> "And then the next thing I knew it was covered. My husband's company Utz Quality Foods was self-funded, and they decided to pay for my treatments."

Hearing the Utz brand's commitment to their employee and his spouse is uplifting and heartwarming.

Cathleen underwent thirty-three proton treatments and six concurrent chemotherapy treatments.

Cathleen's tumor was destroyed by proton radiation, and she had minimal side effects through the concurrent proton and chemotherapy treatments. Yet she still had side effects including nausea and vomiting due to chemotherapy and trigeminal nerve damage from the original tumor, not the proton treatments. She also suffered long-term side effects including bone loss, infections, and holes throughout her sinus cavity due to the death of the tumor. However, many of these side effects were the result of having to receive radiation to the same location twice, due to a recurrence in the jaw. No matter how precise the radiation, having it twice can be damaging, but that's a small price to pay. With protons, Cathleen didn't suffer dry mouth, difficulty swallowing, or severe weight loss that could have required a feeding tube.

Cathleen's patient advocacy continued throughout her journey and still does. During her diagnosis and treatments and thereafter, Cathleen started a blog and shared her experiences with proton radiation and the amazing team at MD Anderson.

"They made me feel like I was one of their children."

Cathleen thought her blog was a good way for people in the community to hear about proton radiation. I had a similar goal when I started my own website about proton radiation. It's through these communications about protons that Cathleen and I feel we are advocating for patients so they can at least ask a doctor:

Are protons right for me?

Cathleen was part of a clinical trial, and she strongly believes, as I do, being part of research is giving a voice to other patients who might need proton radiation.

Cathleen didn't stop there. After her treatments, she chaired the American Cancer Society Relay For Life. I asked her more specifically how she brought patient advocacy to life. She told me:

"It was through the Hero of Hope designation that gave me a voice to share with many different survivor communities. I gave speeches to medical communities at conventions. I shared my story of hope and the power of protons with local news outlets. I wrote articles for local papers. I've been through American Cancer Society's Cancer Action Network, where I am an advocate who has testified before the Austin legislature on cancer-related issues important to the State of Texas. I'm not afraid to share my truth with anyone, anywhere."

When I asked Cathleen what got her through the initial shock of her diagnosis and her experience since then, Cathleen said her faith in God carried her through. It's something she has talked a lot about in her blog.

Prior to being diagnosed, she was mentally and physically strong. That all changed in an instant. Yet, she knew her inability to bear the weight of cancer needed to be given to God and she prayed for God's will to be done:

"The hardest prayer I ever prayed. I asked Him to take it from me. After that I felt such peace and calm throughout the rest of my journey."

Throughout her treatments and thereafter, Cathleen continued to pray verses from the Bible:

"Philippians 4:6–7. 'Do not be anxious about anything, but in every situation, by prayer and petition, with thanksgiving, present your requests to God. And the peace of God which transcends all understanding will guard your hearts and minds in Christ Jesus.'"

I also prayed to God. It helped me cope and face my fears of cancer.

In the article "Cancer: Religion and Spirituality," *Stanford Medicine* authors Andrew W. Kneier, PhD et al. writes that surviving cancer, faith, and religion can provide support in meaningful ways. The article states:

"A person's faith or spirituality provides a means for coping with illness and reaching a deeper kind of inner healing."

Like Cathleen, I had similar experiences with my faith in God. Going to mass and hearing the priests' sermons are my way of connecting to God. There is a universe bigger than me, and my faith in God will carry me through. Before my diagnosis, as much as I could, I attended mass at St. James in Falls Church, Virginia.

One day at mass Father Patrick Posey, our pastor at the time, told a sermon about his faith in God during his earlier days in the ministry. During this time, Father Posey was called by the bishop to discuss his next assignment and found out he was being sent to South America. He told the bishop of course he would go, but he didn't speak Spanish. The bishop told Father Posey he would learn Spanish while in South America and that was the end of that. Father Posey left for South America.

Once he got to South America, Father Posey laid down on the altar and prayed for God to help him learn Spanish. Ultimately, he learned Spanish while fulfilling his role for the community and the church. This story was so inspiring to me and it's one I needed to hear at the time. God works in amazing ways!

At my next proton treatment, I laid on the hard table and visualized myself on the altar of my church. I asked God to heal me. It was a powerful meditation and one that's carried me through treatments and beyond. I consider my faith in God my own form of advocacy. Giving God my fears and anxieties allows me to advocate for myself through my worship of God.

As far as advocacy goes, Cathleen is a role model, someone I look up to, as she's been advocating for many years since her diagnosis and all the while she has battled metastatic disease for the past eight years.

In January of 2015, she was declared to have no evidence of disease (NED) for the first time since her diagnosis. She had fourteen months with NED, but in March of 2016 she was told she had ACC in her liver, which was then surgically removed. Since then, she's had metastatic tumors to her liver and kidney that were treated with ablation procedures.

Then a recurrence in her jaw was treated with SBRT, which is a precise form of high-dose radiation that allows the radiation oncologist to treat cancer in shorter time frames, one to five days, instead of multiple doses over many weeks.

As I write, Cathleen is currently dealing with metastasis (the spread of cancer) in her lungs, liver, peritoneum, omentum, ovary, and sacrum (treated with SRRT). But as Cathleen so beautifully said:

"I know this is all part of His greater plan."

From Cathleen's experiences with cancer and proton radiation, she's dedicated her life to advocacy. Her commitment mirrors that which she witnessed from her doctors at MD Anderson. She told me about a call she received from Dr. Frank:

"A few days after returning home from my thirty-three rounds of proton radiation treatments, Dr. Frank called just to check on me. It wasn't a scheduled appointment, and I wasn't billed for his time. He authentically cared about me."

Dr. Frank sounds incredible, a role model for building relationships with patients, advocating for them, and truly caring about them.

A couple years later, Dr. Frank called her again to see if Cathleen would help advocate as the first patient advocate for the Alliance for Proton Therapy Access, which wasn't yet an official nonprofit. She told me:

"Dr. Frank fought for me. So, now I fight for those who can't."

She's been volunteering her time ever since with the Alliance for Proton Therapy Access where she is an advocate and active member of their board of directors.

One year after her first diagnosis, Cathleen ran her first Relay for Life for the American Cancer Society. Within two days of signing up, she raised $4,000 of the whole event's $15,000. The next year, she became the event lead for the event which raised over $100,000. All total for three years and with the help of her community, they raised $300,000 for the American Cancer Society. During the time of her events, she told everyone she encountered about proton radiation because:

"Protons ultimately saved my life."

Through those initial years and to this day, she's spoken to survivor groups about the power of protons. In 2016, she was a patient advocate speaker at the National Association for Proton Therapy where they discussed insurance denials for proton treatments.

In the spring of 2020 and throughout that year, Cathleen was hospitalized three times due to complications of cancer recurrence and infections. She wasn't allowed to have visitors due to the COVID-19 pandemic, which had escalated in the United States at that time.

During one of her first hospital stays in April of 2020, Cathleen's doctors wanted to discharge her but not send her home. Instead, they wanted to send her to a nursing home to receive treatment and recover because she was on multiple IV antibiotics for a life-threatening infection which required monitoring. They had never sent anyone home on these IV antibiotics for her diagnosis. Yet, they also needed her hospital bed to treat other patients.

Cathleen was by herself. She couldn't have her family at the hospital due to restrictions put in place on visitors during the global pandemic. Cathleen once again had to advocate for herself:

"I'm not leaving this hospital until you figure it out and send me home to my family."

Sure enough, Cathleen stayed in the hospital until they figured out how to send her home with those same IV antibiotics they first said was impossible to do. She hopes other patients who need the same treatment will now benefit from her advocacy.

It broke my heart hearing her story but, at the same time, it showed Cathleen's strength during such a painful time in her life.

Since 2018, Cathleen has been a patient engagement manager at Visiontree Global Health Cloud.

According to their website, Visiontree's mission is to empower patients to improve communication with their provider, maintain their health records, and make better decisions about their health.

As patient engagement manager, Cathleen works directly with thought leaders in the medical community to help create innovative ways to help the company live out its mission. She has done this through the creation of a long-term Cancer Survivorship program, pending Voice For Hope patient platform, quarterly Patient Voice newsletters, and more. She feels like her work is another way to advocate for patients' needs.

They couldn't have a better patient engagement manger than Cathleen.

At home in Austin, Texas, Cathleen enjoys time with her two daughters and husband on the lake, working out, hanging out with friends, and writing her blog which she hopes to turn into a book one day.

As for her health, she is enrolled in a clinical trial, the only available option to treat the widespread metastases in her body. I'm honored to know Cathleen through our work at the Alliance for Proton Therapy Access. I learn from her faith and her advocacy. She is a blessing to everyone who knows her.

One of the prayers that carried Cathleen throughout her journey was:

Jeremiah 29:11: "For I know the plans I have for you, declares the Lord. Plans to prosper you and not to harm you, plans to give you hope and a future."

Yes, God does know His plans for Cathleen. She is an amazing inspiration of hope, love, strength, and determination. The world is a better place because of Cathleen's unwavering desire to help others.

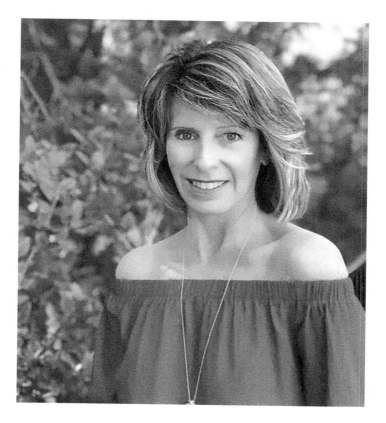

KATE'S STORY
& YOUR LEGAL RIGHTS

"I thought, 'Why am I fighting my insurance company while I am fighting for my life?' Insurance companies don't expect people to fight for their coverage. I fought back."

—KATE WEISSMAN, CANCER SURVIVOR

As I mentioned in a previous chapter, I met Kate through my husband's family who introduced me to her.

When we first chatted about her journey with proton radiation treatment, she told me about the Alliance for Proton Therapy Access and encouraged me to contact the Alliance and share my story with proton radiation, specifically my fight for insurance coverage.

Kate Weissman is courageous and unstoppable. She's also a pillar of strength for cancer survivors. I'm grateful to know Kate and look to her for inspiration.

Here's Kate's incredible story from our interview in the fall of 2020.

Kate is thirty-five years old, a wife, and a PR professional who was born in Boston, raised outside of Philadelphia, and attended Dickinson College. Post-college, Kate lived in Philadelphia, and after working at The Leukemia & Lymphoma Society, she started work at a public relations agency.

In Kate's free time she was a founding member of a nonprofit organization called Fuel the Cure which motivated young professionals to make charitable giving part of their lifestyle. In 2011, Kate moved back to Boston and started working at a different PR agency, Weber Shandwick. She's been there ever since and is now their vice president of integrated project management.

It seems prophetic Kate would land in the field of PR and end up moving back to Boston home of Dana-Farber Cancer Institute, ranked third in the world for cancer care in 2020 by Newsweek. Kate's profession and location in Boston played a role in her proton cancer treatment and ultimate lawsuit with UnitedHealthcare.

Kate was busy living her life and suddenly in October of 2015, Kate was diagnosed with Stage IIB cervical cancer. She underwent thirty rounds of *photon* radiation and six rounds of chemotherapy. It was a brutal treatment course, leaving Kate—an otherwise strong, healthy woman—feeling weak, extremely fatigued, and nauseous.

In the spring of 2016, as part of the follow up protocol, Kate had a PET and CT scans to check for cancer recurrence. The scans showed that while the cancer wasn't on her cervix or in the lymph node, it had spread to her paraaroritc lymph nodes located next to the vertebrae in her lower back.

Kate was devastated.

She underwent surgery to remove the affected lymph nodes. After surgery, her doctors recommended proton radiation. Since the Dana-Farber Cancer Institute didn't have a proton center, Kate was treated at Massachusetts General Hospital (MGH) and the Francis H. Burr Proton Therapy Center. MGH is the academic hospital of Harvard University.

According to a CNN article, both Dana-Farber and MGH doctors believed standard radiation could damage her small intestines, leading to "life-threatening complications later, including ulceration, bleeding, and severe narrowing of the bowel that could cause bowel perforation/rupture, which can be fatal if not treated in a timely fashion." This was according to Dr. Andrea Russo, Kate's primary oncologist at the time. It could also "damage her kidneys and cause long-term bone marrow issues." The same article states:

> "On April 6, 2016, UnitedHealthcare denied coverage, contending that proton beam therapy (PBT) is experimental or investigational or unproven."

Despite the army of support for Kate's case, (UHC) denied approval for proton radiation treatment and instead approved standard radiation treatment IMRT.

Kate's medical team kept pushing for coverage while Kate and her husband Matt took their fight to the next level with an impressive coalition of experts.

Six oncologists advocated on Kate's behalf, including five who also teach at Harvard Medical School and a sixth who was once named among America's top doctors by Newsweek. Aides in the offices of Senators Elizabeth Warren and Ed Markey also pressed UHC about covering Kate's proton treatment.

Kate told me:

> *"I remember calling the insurance company from my chemo chair, begging them to approve my treatment. As I was battling for my life, I was also battling UnitedHealthcare."*

Kate's physician, Whitfield B. Growdon, MD, explained to Kate he could see both sides of her case from the viewpoint of UHC and his own as to why he prescribed protons. In a CNN article he explained:

"In UHC denials, there is little evidence to support proton beam therapy for cervical cancer. We don't have randomized trials, nor Kate are we ever going to have randomized trials for this. Finding one hundred patients with cervical cancer that spread to the paraaortic lymph nodes, fifty of them for standard radiation and fifty for proton beam therapy is just not plausible or feasible. We need to be innovative with our care as long as we fervently believe we can do it safely, that we're not going to hurt you."

It frustrates me as to why Kate's case got denied, yet others like mine got approved.

According to the *Boston Globe*, a spokesperson for UHC told the reporter in an email:

> *"UnitedHealthcare bases its medical policies and coverage decisions—including for proton beam therapy—on the prevailing published clinical and scientific evidence."*
>
> —MARIA GORDON SHYDLO, UNITEDHEALTHCARE

But to Dr. Growdon's point, it's next to impossible to provide this type of research for Kate's specific diagnosis as finding patients who have this same diagnosis and then juxtapose them in a randomized clinical trial isn't feasible. But this is the gist of the UHC denial.

It seems so unjust that a doctor prescribed Kate proton radiation, knowing this was the safest and best choice for her, but the insurance company decided otherwise without even meeting Kate.

Kate's case was ultimately reviewed, denied, and appealed six times—to no avail. Denying coverage for this reason is a disgrace, yet this happens day in and day out across the United States with various insurance providers.

Kate urgently needed to be treated.

Weeks went by and in May of 2016, Kate's parents offered to help. They wired $95,000 to MGH from their 401K retirement plan so Kate could immediately be treated. Although grateful, this was extremely stressful for Kate.

When we talked about Kate's difficult experience with UHC, she told me:

> *"My mental health also suffered during proton therapy because I was fighting with my insurance company to cover my treatments. Ultimately, my parents paid for it so that was emotionally very difficult, and it was hard to navigate fighting with the insurance and for my life at the same time."*

Kate was successfully treated with proton radiation in May of 2016. She recovered well with minimal side effects. She took time to heal both physically and mentally and then she stood up and fought again.

Kantor & Kantor LLP explained in a press release which was picked up across the media:

"On March 26, 2019, Kate Weissman filed a class action lawsuit to challenge what she alleges to be UnitedHealthcare's unfair and deceptive policies and procedures for determining whether a prescribed treatment or medication is medically necessary (utilization review). Kate Weissman alleges that UnitedHealthcare's utilization review process is skewed toward the denial of coverage based upon inadequate internal medical policies placed in the hands of unqualified medical directors."

It takes a lot of time, energy, and bravery to fight back. Kate told me she and Matt felt called to do it. I had a similar feeling when I ended treatment. I wanted to find other patients stories that fought back and won against their insurance provider to be able to instill hope for patients navigating this horrific and stressful process.

Around the same time in April, 2019 in southern Florida, ThinkAdvisor.com reported that a judge had recused himself from a case of a prostate cancer patient seeking to sue UHC with a class action lawsuit over a denial of coverage for proton radiation. United States District Judge Robert Scola's friend Robert Cole was treated with proton radiation. His friend's treatments were declined by UHC, so he paid $150,000 out of pocket to receive treatment. His friend told Judge Scola that UHC agreed to reimburse him "only upon threat of litigation."

In the article, the same spokesperson who commented on Kate's case, Maria Gordon Shydlo, at UHC said pretty much the same thing she'd stated for Kate's case:

"UHC bases its medical policies and coverage decisions—including for proton beam therapy—on the prevailing published clinical and scientific evidence."

Judge Scola, states in the article;

> "To deny a patient this treatment, if it is available, is immoral and barbaric."

Along with Kate, Robert Cole and another patient also decided to sue UHC.

For Kate and Matt, their lawsuit is about justice for Kate, Matt, and her family, and for those she doesn't know. It's about paying it forward and creating positive change in the healthcare system.

When I met Kate, I felt guilty my treatments were approved and hers weren't. I wasn't fighting cancer twice, just once. We both had UHC health insurance. We don't know the similarities or differences in our plans. We live in different states. But somehow, I imagine these variables matter to UHC in how they determined to cover our cases.

It makes me think, are we simply viewed by UHC as policy holders and not valued customers or, *better yet, patients in need?*

In my case, did UHC evaluate my heart and determine that was worth sparing and approved proton radiation after I appealed the denials for my case? But Kate's vital organs weren't worth sparing?

This makes me sick.

After Kate and I met in 2019, I agreed to talk to her attorney, Mr. Rich Collins, Senior Trial Attorney at Callahan & Blaine. I wanted to share my story and case as I thought maybe it would help Kate.

Since I knew Rich, I reached out to him to ask if I could interview him and Mr. Tim Rozelle, an Associate at Kantor & Kantor LLP, for this book. Both Tim and Rich are part of the Proton Therapy Law Coalition which Tim started in 2019. The coalition of lawyers was created to bring physicians, patient advocates, patients, and attorneys across the country to challenge proton beam therapy insurance denials.

I asked Rich and Tim:

What should a patient know about legal representation if they are denied proton treatment by their insurance company?

Both attorneys typically work with clients on a **contingency fee** basis. This means their attorney's fees are contingent upon their success in getting a favorable resolution—settlement or court judgment. If a case is successful, the attorneys may be able to obtain their attorney's fees from the defendants but, if not, a certain contingency percentage written into a client retainer agreement will govern how much of the settlement or court judgment will go toward attorney's fees. According to Rich, typically, this figure is in the ballpark of forty percent.

NEXT, DOES THE TYPE OF INSURANCE PLAN MATTER WHEN SEEKING PROTON RADIATION?

According to Rich:

"At the root of all the disputes with the insurance there's a piece of paper, a contract. And that's what's supposed to govern. The process starts with getting my arms around what the plan is, and then my head around what the rules of engagement are as the first step to help my clients."

Tim Rozelle works with clients whose insurance is governed by the Employee Retirement Security Act (ERISA).

Tim weighed in:

"Unlike bad faith insurance cases in certain state jurisdictions, ERISA places certain limits on the remedies a claimant (client) can seek because of a wrongful denial of benefits. Typically, ERISA limits potential recovery to the verified amount of a claimant's out-of-pocket, private pay costs for treatment. ERISA also requires a claimant submit an exhaustive and thorough set of appeals prior to filing suit. This set of appeals and the documents, information, and data submitted along with these submissions to the Plan administrator or insurance company, constitutes the 'administrative record.'"

Attorneys like Tim help patients understand the law and what's needed before deciding whether to sue.

Tim and Rich are so professional and are there to support and provide resources for patients if their case for insurance coverage for protons is denied.

As for Kate's lawsuit, in March of 2021, Reuters reported Kate, Richard Coles, and another case filed against UHC were allowed to proceed in court. United States District Judge Allison Burroughs denied UHC's motion to dismiss the three lawsuits that alleged UHC "deceptively and unfairly administered their ERISA plans by refusing to cover Proton Beam Radiation Therapy (PBRT)…because it is more expensive than more traditional cancer treatments."

As Rich Collins stated in litigation-update.com on Kate Weissman's, Zachary Ritzzuto's, and Roslyn Gonzalez's cases:

"We have some of the world's most renowned radiation oncologists who have recommended proton beam therapy for their patients, explaining in detail for the insurance company why it's medically necessary and why the safety and quality of their patients' lives are at stake, only to have a medical director for the insurance company overrule their recommendation. When the denial letter is peeled back and it's revealed who the doctor is that made the determination, in each of these cases, **it was not a board-certified radiation oncologist**."

I'm so proud of Kate for pushing forward for justice not only for her family but for patients in the months and years ahead.

Kate's final thoughts on proton radiation:

> *"I'm confident proton radiation saved me from health complications in my vital organs. Because of protons, I'm able to live a healthy life post cancer."*

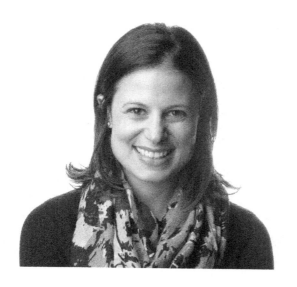

PART THREE:
LEGISLATE

HOW & WHY I SHOULD
TALK TO MY LEGISLATOR

"Legislators are talking to constituents of lobbyists all day long, and they're getting reams of paper, the things that stand out for them are the stories. It's that simple. It's very powerful."

—MOLLY DANIELS, EXECUTIVE DIRECTOR,
ALLIANCE FOR PROTON THERAPY ACCESS

In November of 2003, Nancy Cappello, PhD, had her annual mammogram. She was told everything was normal. Six weeks later at her annual exam, her doctor felt a ridge in her right breast. She sent Nancy to get another mammogram and an ultrasound. The ultrasound picked up a 2.3 cm lesion, but the mammogram came back normal. Nancy was diagnosed with Stage IIIC breast cancer after having two normal mammograms. Because she had dense breast tissue, the mammogram couldn't pick up the cancer. Cancer presents white on a mammogram and so does the dense breast tissue, so it was more difficult to detect. Nancy's story is shared on the Areyoudense.org website where she described how she found out she had dense breasts and further, why this is so important to know.

Finding out she had dense breasts at the same time she was diagnosed with cancer upset Nancy so much she decided to research about dense breast tissue. What she found was startling. For almost a decade before her diagnosis, according to the website:

> *"Six major studies with over 42,000 women concluded by supplementing a mammogram with an ultrasound increases detection from 48 percent to 97 percent for women with dense tissue."*

It was then that Nancy, together with her husband Joe, decided they needed do something about the lack of knowledge and communication about dense breasts. Joe and Nancy created a grassroots movement called Are You Dense Inc. and Are You Dense Advocacy. In October of 2009, Connecticut was the first state to mandate legislation for breast density notification. By March of 2019, the FDA announced the Mammography Quality Standards Act, requiring all fifty states and United States territories to include patient notification from mammogram reports and summaries, which includes information on breast density.

In 2012, I remember getting a letter from the radiology center telling me I had dense breasts. I researched the topic of dense breasts and found Nancy's story. I was inspired by her ability to take a tragic diagnosis and create change. I remember telling my friends, mom, and sister about breast density, asking: "Do you know if you are dense?" Nancy's movement resonated with me.

Sadly, Nancy died in November of 2018 from a blood disorder associated with the side effects from her cancer treatments, but by then more than half of the states had legislation around breast density notification. I hadn't thought about legislation for proton radiation access and prior authorization approvals until Dr. Eblan mentioned it. **He knew I was stressed but said if I wanted to advocate for change, I could reach out to my congressman.**

Finding out I had cancer and seeing the inefficient and broken insurance system simultaneously play out, I was both fearful and furious. My insurance was seemingly holding proton radiation to a different standard than traditional radiation, calling it "medically unnecessary." Many patients even heard the word "experimental."

Prior to treatment, when I was on the phone with United-Healthcare begging to talk to the doctors who denied my claim, I was told I couldn't speak to the UHC doctors. I got even more stressed. Then the icing on the cake when the UHC representative told me I could fax an appeal to the insurance company over the denial of my treatment coverage. I felt let down as a customer. I wouldn't describe my encounter as excellent, good, or even fair. It was awful.

I thought a lot about Dr. Eblan's advice around advocacy as I heard more and more insurance denials and appeals for proton happened all the time. I lived in Virginia, but was being treated in Maryland, so Dr. Eblan said my case might be affected by the location of my cancer treatment center.

I learned in 2017 that the state legislature in Virginia had already passed legislation that might have approved my treatments quicker had I been treated in Virginia. According to the website law.lis.virginia.gov:

> "*Notwithstanding the provisions of § 38.2-3419, each policy, contract, or plan issued or provided by a carrier that provides coverage for cancer therapy* **shall not hold proton radiation therapy to a higher standard of clinical evidence** *for decisions regarding coverage under the policy, contract, or plan than is applied for decisions regarding coverage of other types of radiation therapy treatment.*"

Yet in 2020, Coach Rivera was treated in Fairfax, Virginia and his **initial** prior authorization was declined for proton treatment. Coach's case got overturned on the same day, but why did it get declined to begin with?

During treatments, I met patients in the waiting room at the Maryland Proton Treatment Center (MPTC) and thereafter who gratefully had no trouble getting insurance to pay for proton radiation, with one caveat—these patients were routinely Medicare or Medicaid, some with AARP supplements. In general, according to the medicare.org website, Medicare will pay for most medically necessary radiation therapies whether inpatient or outpatient. Each patient's plan determines out of pocket estimates. This is a good thing!

However, the words "medically necessary" stand out to me even on the Medicare website as a way to treat proton radiation differently, create a loophole by claiming it medically unnecessary when reviewing a prior authorization for approval.

Therefore, federal legislation is needed to change the prior authorization process for what attorney Rich Collins of Callahan & Blaine in our interview called "proton parody," where proton radiation won't be held to a higher standard to photon treatment. Proton and photon therapies will be equal in the eyes of the insurance providers. Yet, this legislation was created in Virginia and people are still getting denied on the first prior authorization request.

Dr. Eblan treats patients in the state of Virginia and he said during our interview in the winter of 2020:

> *"For certain liver cancers, I still have to fight with some insurance companies to get this approved, which is really infuriating."*

In the summer of 2019, about fourteen months after treatment ended, I decided to reach out to my congressman and share my story about prior authorization and proton radiation. I wasn't intimidated, but I thought I had to be an expert on insurance claims or the approval process, and I wasn't an expert on either. I was a patient who cared and felt I wanted to make a difference so others wouldn't go through what I went through.

By this time, I decided to share my story, I was a volunteer proton champion at the Alliance for Proton Therapy Access. I asked Molly Daniels, the Executive Director at the Alliance, for her help and suggestions. She said the same thing then as she did when I interviewed her for this book:

"People think they can't write a letter or visit their congressman unless they know every single detail of the issue, and that's just not true. They just need to tell their story."

In August of 2019, I emailed Congressman Don Beyer's office of the 8th District of Virginia. Congress is in recess in August, so I gave it a few weeks, and emailed again and still didn't receive a response. I called the office in the fall, and someone gave me a new email address, so I emailed that person.

Then on January 16, 2020, I finally heard back from someone who apologized for the lack of response. They'd had a staffing change and my email somehow got lost. By January 22, 2020, I heard back from one of Congressman Beyer's senior legislative staffers:

> *"Great! Denise, are you a constituent of the Congressman? I'm trying to understand the background on why you are talking with our office."*

Staying patient and persistent, a few days later I explained who I was and told this person a little bit more about my story which I had included on all the emails I had sent before. I said I'd been trying to talk to someone in the office since August of 2019, five months ago. She offered to meet with me on February 13, 2020, and I booked the appointment to meet at the Longworth Office Building in Washington, DC. I went with my husband and a fellow breast cancer survivor, Jillian Benstein.

Heading into the appointment with Congressman Beyer's senior staffer, we didn't know what to expect and that's probably a good thing. Jillian and I told Congressman Beyer's staffer our stories and she listened, then said there wasn't much she could do because it was an election year and things slowed down.

She mentioned a healthcare bill going forward to Congress in May, but other than that, she seemed almost bored with our stories. Jillian and I picked up on this and we ended our meeting within about thirty minutes. We were so disappointed.

On the way home, we tossed around ideas of why our stories weren't impactful. We thought maybe the staff must see a lot of people and our cancer stories were just one of many. Yet I couldn't help drawing a parallel to the thousands of guests I served and met through my career at Marriott International. If I didn't create a welcoming space for our guests, it was unacceptable. I liked it that way, as all of us on the team at Marriott were held to the same standard of service excellence. Apparently, this doesn't apply in government, even though the men and women in Congress are there to serve their constituents. That model didn't pencil out in my first visit to Congressman Beyer's office.

But I haven't given up hope legislation can change the prior authorization process for healthcare providers and patients.

Since 2017, the American Medical Association (AMA) has worked with seventeen state and specialty medical societies, other healthcare organizations, and patients to develop best practices for prior authorization research and reform. There are webinars and short videos for healthcare providers on best practices within the current system and ways for improvement toward an optimal and efficient system for all.

In tandem, the AMA created a grassroots advocacy effort to change the legislation for prior authorization approvals. Patients, physicians, and employers can share their stories to affect positive change in legislature at the fixpriorauth.org website. I signed the petition and encourage other patients to share their story if they are comfortable in doing so.

A YouTube video titled "Prior Authorization is a Nightmare" illustrates how frustrating the process can be for physicians and patients and why legislation is needed. As mentioned, this process affects patients seeking proton radiation, but also affects patients seeking insurance approval for procedures, scans, medicine, and more. The video sums up the prior authorization process and need for reform.

"It cripples my patients; it cripples my medical practice."

—MATTHEW GRIERSON, MD, PSYCHIATRY

"Prior authorization is just a disaster both for the physicians, but more so for the patients."

—JERRY KENNETT, MD, CARDIOLOGY

"It frustrates physicians endlessly. I would hope patients know physicians are on the same team. I encourage patients to sign the petition."

—BARBARA L. MCANENY, MD, PRESIDENT OF ONCOLOGY 2018–2019

Since then, in June of 2020 the AMA released results of a survey and a statement on the current state of prior authorization:

"Prior authorization continues to interfere with patient care and can lead to adverse clinical consequences with

16 percent of physicians reporting the process has led to a patient's hospitalization."

If that's not concerning enough, physicians also reported frustration over the lack of progress with legislative efforts, despite a consensus statement signed by healthcare organizations such as the AMA, Blue Cross Blue Shield Association, and four other organizations. However, it's clear the AMA will continue to push for this legislation. I'm so grateful for their hard work and efforts and I'm just as proud of patients who reached out to tell their stories.

I asked Kim Jones, an attorney at Aulsbrook Law Firm in Arlington, Texas, about her experience with prior authorization denials for proton radiation:

What would you say to legislators about proton therapy or the prior authorization process if you had the chance to talk to them?

Kim told me she will have the chance to talk to legislators as she's a civil attorney working with her local constituent to write legislation that will hold proton therapy treatment to the same standard as other radiation treatments:

"What I'm hoping to do legislatively, is what Oklahoma has done to close the loophole saying insurers can't hold proton therapy to a higher standard. We can't mandate the insurance companies to cover it, that wouldn't be constitutional. But we can say, 'You're manipulating the system, you're using this loophole, we need to close the loophole.'"

Kim is so inspiring! She beat cancer and now she's working on legislation to create proton parity and close the loophole so other patients don't go through what we went through.

According to leg.colorod.gov in February of 2021, Democratic Representative Karen McCormick and Republican Representative Matt Soper proposed a bill which would:

> *"Prohibit health benefit plans that provides coverage for cancer treatment from applying a higher standard of clinical evidence for coverage of proton beam therapy than the health benefit plan applies for other radiation therapy treatment."*

When I heard this news at our monthly meeting at the Alliance for Proton Therapy Access, I was thrilled! Not only because this adds to the list of five states that have passed similar bills (Oregon, Virginia, Oklahoma, Tennessee, and Mississippi), but it proves patients and providers who have spoken have been heard. Finally, it's a bi-partisan bill that's been put forward.

As of March 10, 2021, the legislation has been postponed indefinitely, but I hope it will be passed.

On Saturday, June 26, 2021, I received an email from the Proton Therapy Law Coalition with an update from an article featured on The Lund Report, "Senate Approves Bill To Ease Barriers To Therapy For Prostate Cancer." The article summarized the Oregon lawmakers approved Senate Bill 2 A which:

"Prohibits insurers from imposing prior authorization or other utilization review requirements on coverage for proton beam therapy for prostate cancer that are more restrictive than prior authorization or utilization review requirements applied to coverage of radiation therapy."

Hooray! This is such an exciting first step for prostate cancer patients and hopefully more can be done for other cancer patients seeking proton therapy in Oregon.

This bill was put forth by Senator Bill Hansell R-Athena as he benefited from proton treatment twenty-one years ago. Senator Hansell said:

"But it required jumping through too many insurance hoops. If an Oregonian and their doctor decide proton beam therapy is the best treatment option, this bill will make it easier to access."

The article went on to say that in 2019 "the Legislature passed Senate Bill 740, which required insurers to cover proton beam therapy in the same way they cover radiation therapy. But that bill had a loophole which allowed insurers to put more extensive prior authorization conditions in place (for protons)." The new bill would prohibit this for happening, at least for prostate cancer.

There are countless stories of people who have spoken up and advocated for change. Because of their activism, laws have been created such as the Mammography Quality Standards Act and The Women's Health and Cancer Rights Act (WHCRA) of 1998. WHRCA is a federal law that provides protections to patients who choose to have breast reconstruction in connection with a mastectomy. My plastic surgeon, Ariel Rad, PhD, MD, told me about this act when we first met to discuss my mastectomy plans. He told me insurance had to cover the cost of reconstruction as it's the law.

The law began in 1997, according to Wikipedia, when Janet Franquet was told by her insurance provider that her mastectomy was cosmetic and not "medically necessary." Dr. Wider, Janet's doctor, performed her mastectomy reconstruction for free, but he was so upset, he contacted several legislators to create change. Senator Alfonse D'Amato became one of the most vocal and addressed Congress, saying:

> "Mr. President, I decided that I would give Mrs. Franquet's insurance company a call. When I spoke with the medical director, he told me that 'replacement of a breast is not **medically necessary**. This is not a bodily function and therefore cannot and should not be replaced.' I ask you, Mr. President, how many other Janet Franquets are out there? Will they be lucky enough to have a Dr. Wider to take care of them?"

I find myself ready to present to Congress or the President to seek change within the prior authorization process and access to proton radiation through creating proton parity as Senate Bill 2A has done in Oregon. After all, how many patients right now are seeking access to proton and continually being denied? I can't imagine how many. We must speak up if we want to see change.

KIM'S STORY OF LYMPHOMA & LEGISLATURE

"Keep fighting. That's the best advice I've got. It's so hard but keep persevering. It might not work out, but we don't have to make it easy on the insurance companies. We can at least make a point they can't just keep treating people like this and walking all over us. Keep fighting."

—KIM JONES, CANCER SURVIVOR

Kim and I also met at the Alliance for Proton Therapy Access where she is a volunteer and advocate. In the fall of 2020, I interviewed Kim.

Here's her story.

Kim Jones, twenty-five years old and an attorney at Aulsbrook Law Firm in Arlington, Texas, works primarily on personal injury and wrongful death cases. In her work she deals with auto insurance or commercial policies for trucking collision cases. She also handles premises liability cases where someone has been injured or killed due to a hazardous condition on another's property.

Kim is very passionate about her work and believes strongly in protecting her clients and getting them compensation when they are injured and at a low point in their lives. As such, she spends a lot of her time fighting with insurance companies to get her clients what they deserve.

One day in December of 2017, she was fiddling with her necklace at work. She noticed a lump in her neck and thought, *Hmmm, maybe I should get this checked out?*

She went to her primary care physician (PCP) who ordered tests, including a CT scan. Days later her scans came back, and she got a phone call from her PCP's physician assistant (PA) on a Friday asking her to come in on the following Monday to review the CT in-person. Kim told me:

"I think any time a doctor asks to deliver news in-person there is sort of a sinking feeling in the pit of a person's stomach. I was in the car with my boss at the time, but I begged the PA to not make me wait and worry myself sick all weekend."

Finally, the PA got permission to tell Kim over the phone that they found more tumors than just the one on her neck which had been her initial concern. The PA told Kim she needed an immediate consultation with an oncologist who would take over from there.

Kim was still in the car heading back to the office with her boss, so she asked him if she could meet her husband Carson and head home. Kim met Carson in a parking lot and, as they drove home, she told him she might have cancer. She felt detached from her own words when she told her boss but with Carson, she broke down crying. It didn't feel real.

Kim moved through more appointments and then her tumor was biopsied next.

It was negative, no cancer! Kim and Carson celebrated, what a huge relief!

Kim's oncologist recommended a second CT scan six months later, just to be sure, and keep a watch on the area.

By then, the tumor had grown and Kim started getting that same sinking feeling in her stomach. Kim started getting symptoms like itching feet (Hodgkin's itch) and fatigue creeped in and had gotten worse. Kim's family stayed optimistic, but it started settling in—she could have cancer.

Six months went by and after the CT, Kim's doctor scheduled surgery to remove the lymph node in her neck to get a larger sample size of pathology from a new biopsy. The surgeon seemed optimistic it could be benign and offered to let Kim know more about what the surgeon found when she woke up from surgery.

The surgery was more complex than expected, and the lymph node was larger than they thought. When Kim woke up, her surgeon recommended she go back to see her oncologist. Kim told me:

"It may have been the anesthesia, but it seemed like the nurses were avoiding eye contact with me when I asked them if it was cancer."

A few days later, after Christmas, Kim braced herself for bad news. She thought they would have let her know right away if it wasn't cancer.

I can't imagine how stressful those days, weeks, and months must have been. Yet in some ways, Kim's worst battle was ahead of her.

At the oncologist's office, she finally heard the words, "You have cancer."

Kim was diagnosed with Stage II Hodgkin's lymphoma.

According to Cancercenter.com, the website for Cancer Treatment Centers of America, Hodgkin's lymphoma develops in the lymphocytes, which are cells in the lymphatic system—a network of vessels, nodes, and organs. The lymphatic system's primary role is to help fight infection by filtering waste and toxins from the body. The spleen, thymus, tonsils, and bone marrow form part of the lymphatic system along with 650 lymph nodes scattered throughout the body. Two cells make up the lymphocytes in the lymphatic system, B-cells and T-cells. B-cells are more likely to mutate and cause "liquid cancer," non-solid such as Hodgkin's lymphoma.

Cancer.net explains Stage II Hodgkin's lymphoma means there is either:

- Cancer in two or more lymph node regions on the same side of the diaphragm.

Or

- The cancer involves one organ and regional lymph nodes with or without cancer in other lymph node regions on the same side of the diaphragm.

Further on Cancercenter.com, roughly 170,000 blood cancer diagnoses such as leukemia, myeloma, and Hodgkin's lymphoma are diagnosed each year. Unlike these disease types, most cancers are solid and made from mutated cells that grow out of control and into tumors found in breast, lung, prostate, and colorectal. About one million cases of these solid cancer cases are diagnosed each year in the United States.

After hearing the news, Kim and her mom stood in the parking lot of the doctor's office. It was a nice sunny day outside and they weren't sure where to go or what to do from there.

In the parking lot, Kim thought about movies where it cuts to the next scene. She envisioned herself starting chemotherapy, but she still had another two or three weeks to go for fertility treatments, port placement, and surgery, and then she would begin chemotherapy.

Kim went to lunch with her mom, and spent the rest of the day with her parents. When Carson got home from work, he took her out to dinner at one of her favorite local restaurants. They held hands and he constantly reassured Kim they would get through it.

Then they started embryo harvesting and all the preparation work before chemo.

Kim remembers looking at herself in the mirror over those two or three weeks before chemo and thinking how she didn't actually look any different than she had before finding out she had cancer. It definitely took a while for the news to really sink in. A lot of mornings she woke up thinking it was a bad dream, but it would all come flooding back. I felt the same way when I was diagnosed, except I didn't have any symptoms, just cancer growing in my breast.

After a series of doctor appointments, Kim started chemotherapy in January of 2018, and before she finished in March of 2018, it was rough. Eventually, she learned to accept the diagnosis, especially after losing her hair.

Through it all, Carson was her rock. He attended every chemo and medical appointment with Kim. He was a pillar of strength, love, and support. He was in school at the time and took a semester off just to take care of his beloved wife. She told me in our interview:

"I can't express in words how much his love and support meant to me."

There were intermittent days Kim just couldn't work, especially the day or two after chemo. She learned to get by with naps and a flexible work schedule. Some nights her insomnia was terrible, which was most likely caused by side effects of the steroids and chemotherapy. When insomnia kept her awake her thoughts would wander to her chemo treatments. Were they working? Was she healing? So many nights, she checked her emails and started back at work until she would get so tired she'd go back to bed. Always keeping others in mind, Kim delayed delivering her emails through Microsoft Outlook so she wouldn't disrupt her colleague's sleep at 3:00 or 4:00 a.m.

When Kim finished chemotherapy, she was sent for her consultation with a radiation oncologist. Like many patients who finish chemo, Kim was extremely fatigued and nauseas. To say it was rough is an understatement.

At this point, Kim was referred to a radiation oncologist who started talking about her plan for radiation. The conversation started with photon radiation (IMRT) and that was that. So, Kim asked:

"Well are there other types of radiation where there are fewer side effects?"

Kim didn't feel good about the plan for IMRT, so she spoke up and asked about other options. She knew deep down she had to keep asking questions. She couldn't take the doctor's recommendation as the plan as she faced the possibility of being on a feeding tube as a side effect as a result of IMRT treatment to her esophagus and salivary glands.

On top of the risk of being on a feeding tube, her doctors said she might lose her sense of taste, at least for a little while, or it could be potentially permanent. Her salivary glands would be impacted which could impair her ability to produce saliva. Photon radiation would also put her at a higher risk of heart disease, heart attack, breast cancer, lung cancer, and secondary issues from chest radiation. The exit dose with photon radiation would have gone through Kim's spinal cord, increasing the risk of myeloma, a cancer of the bone marrow.

These are major side effects and worth consideration when contemplating treatment plans.

As all this unfolded, Kim continued asking questions. She knew each side effect was a possibility, but what if that possibility became a reality? She asked her doctors:

"Is there something better? Is there something else we can do? This seems a little extreme."

After her appointment, Kim started to research radiation treatment options. She Googled the terms, and through her research, learned about proton radiation at MD Anderson and other places closer to her in Texas.

MD Anderson was the first to respond to Kim's inquiry, but it wasn't the closest to her home. Yet, several friends had recommended it from personal reference. So, Kim decided to make an appointment for a second opinion where she heard right away at this first appointment:

"You're a great candidate for proton therapy. You may get a little bit of a sunburn, and have other mild side effects, a cough, fatigue, sore throat, but you will be good to go."

Kim thought… what a night and day difference between the potential side effects. She decided to go with the team at MD Anderson and her records were immediately transferred to her new radiation oncologist.

Kim's doctor warned her many times insurance doesn't approve the treatment on the first try through the prior authorization process, but they were hopeful it would be approved. Her doctor sent her case in for prior authorization to her insurance, BlueCross BlueShield.

Then the stress began.

Immediately, her insurance provider denied her case.

Kim finished chemo in March of 2018 and was supposed to start radiation within a couple of weeks from that time. So, Kim's physician appealed her case and asked for an expedited case review so she could start treatment. Kim's case was unique. She was young, twenty-five, when she was diagnosed. Traditional photon radiation even with IMRT had potential side effects as mentioned earlier, and her doctor also included in the letter the fact photon radiation would pass through the body so she would receive radiation exposure to her chest and her spinal cord.

Since one of the tumors was in the anterior mediastinum, or in laymen's terms, the space between her sternum and heart, this was a big issue. This increased Kim's future risk for stroke, heart attack, and heart failure with traditional radiation. Her doctor again thought age would play in her favor as she had so many years of life ahead of her.

So, her physician laid all the facts of her case to BlueCross BlueShield.

They denied her case again.

Then her doctor appealed again.

Next BlueCross BlueShield sent her case for an outside review to a company called eviCore who explains part of their services to patients and providers on their website:

> "A company committed to advancing healthcare management through intelligent care—and enabling **better outcomes** for patients, providers, and health plans."

eviCore denied Kim's case.

Interesting. I would like to talk to the leaders of eviCore about how they define "better outcomes." Is the potential of radiation exposure to the heart and spinal cord a better outcome? How about the possibility Kim would have a risk of going on a feeding tube as a result of traditional photon radiation IMRT? Is that a better outcome? Maybe it's a better outcome cost-wise for the insurers? Her risk of secondary cancers, like lung cancer and breast cancer, would also be increased due to the unnecessary radiation going through her body from IMRT. I wonder how this can be called a "better outcome?"

By then weeks had gone by and Kim wasn't in treatment.

Kim was determined to get her treatments covered. As a lawyer dedicated to winning cases and fighting insurance companies day in and day out to protect her clients and get them what they deserved, suddenly she found herself fighting in the same way—this time for herself.

Backed against a wall, Kim prepared her strategy and next steps. She considered appealing to the Texas Department of

Insurance (TDI) or contacting the media. She even thought about doing both. She wasn't giving up.

Coincidentally, Kim had mutual friends who were friends with her local state representative. Kim's friends jumped right in. One of them had the personal cell phone number of the local representative and called him and said:

"You've got to do something on this quickly."

Kim's doctors and her team at MD Anderson put together an expert appeals packet, and even had side-by-side photos showing what photon IMRT would potentially do to Kim's body versus proton therapy's effect. MD Anderson came to Kim's aid by having a professional who was both a lawyer and a doctor work on her appeal. Kim's case was strong from both a legal and medical aspect.

But Kim's an attorney too, and she wanted to stay involved in her own case. She told me:

"Even though I was tired from chemotherapy, I spent hours researching, using my legal expertise, to research my own case. It was exhausting, but I had to do it. I had to fight back and try and help."

Then Kim's oncologist called and said she might need to go back into chemotherapy, because it had been too long without continuation of treatment. She was devastated and angry—on a roller coaster of emotions that all stemmed from the insurance provider's policies and procedures. This is so unjust.

Kim submitted her case to her local constituent and then it was submitted to TDI.

Through this process, Kim finally got a neutral third party radiation oncologist to review the file through TDI. She described:

> *"And when they reviewed it, the independent radiation oncologist agreed with my doctors at MD Anderson and said this was medically necessary and **should not have been denied**."*

TDI overturned BlueCross BlueShield's decision, and forced them to pay for her treatments.

Through it all, Kim's proton radiation treatments were delayed for two months while her case went back and forth, through the prior authorization denial, appeal, denial, appeal, third party review, and then finally her state representative stepped in and TDI overturned her case.

All this occurred while Kim was struggling to receive treatment—at the mercy of the insurance company who was ultimately blocking payment until potentially she would give up.

But Kim didn't give up.

I didn't either.

After Kim's treatments were approved, she got started right away on two weeks of proton therapy. Since the treatment center was five hours from her home, she reserved a hotel room and her husband joined her for each proton treatment.

Kim's treatments went well. Like the Maryland Proton Treatment Center (MPTC), MD Anderson also lets patients pick their own music selection during treatments. Kim decided to go with Bob Marley and try to relax by taking slow breaths.

She would also meditate and chant "don't worry be happy" to get through.

I asked Kim about her mental health. How did she handle the stress before, during, and after treatment?

Her oncologist recommended psychotherapy during Kim's treatments and thereafter. Kim wasn't sure how she felt about it, but it was free through the Rutledge Foundation at the oncologist's office. Kim thought, it's free so she might as well go.

Kim told me the therapy was so helpful and still is:

"I can't recommend therapy enough. I learned meditation and ways to calm my mind naturally, it's so worth it."

I had anxiety with my cancer diagnosis and treatment, too. It's almost unavoidable I think to some degree. I learned through therapy at MPTC that I could either deal with the emotions now, or at some point in my life the diagnosis and treatments would come crashing down on me and I could have a break down. So, I saw a therapist too.

I also learned how to meditate, which is one of the biggest gifts from cancer. I don't use that language lightly, but cancer does give gifts.

After chemo and proton radiation, Kim had fatigue. She had swelling and gained weight from the steroids used during her chemo treatments.

She had hair loss, and then after radiation it grew back curly, and that was another adjustment.

It was close to two years after treatment when Kim thought:

"I need to go back to therapy."

In January of 2020, Kim went back to therapy and has been going back ever since. She faces different concerns now: *What will the future bring? Will I get cancer again?*

Most cancer patients like Kim and me also follow a routine of repeat visits with our medical team. We get more scans looking for cancer. So naturally, right before getting the scans, there's more worry: Will they find cancer again?

Knowing Kim from our volunteer work, I would have never dreamt her story was this difficult. She's so graceful, professional, and inspiring in so many ways. She's brave and wise. Here's Kim's advice regarding advocacy:

> *"If you have a lump at any age, you should take it seriously. If you don't feel good, you've got to keep speaking up. Three years leading up to my own diagnosis, I knew people in*

college and law school who were so tired. But my fatigue was different. Each time the doctors tested me for mono. If it's negative, you're good to go. But a lot of the symptoms of my cancer mimicked the symptoms of mono. And so, it's really tough, finding or getting doctors to take it seriously at a young age."

Kim's advice on advocating with the physicians:

"You've got to speak up. Ask questions. Bring someone with you to ask questions too."

I asked Kim: **What would you like to tell legislators about what you went through with prior authorization?**

Kim said:

"Listen to your constituents and cancer patients. I'm writing the legislation myself and looking for support from our legislators. If we're going to have change, we have to drive the change we want to see."

Wow! After all she's been through, she's thinking of others and is making a difference.

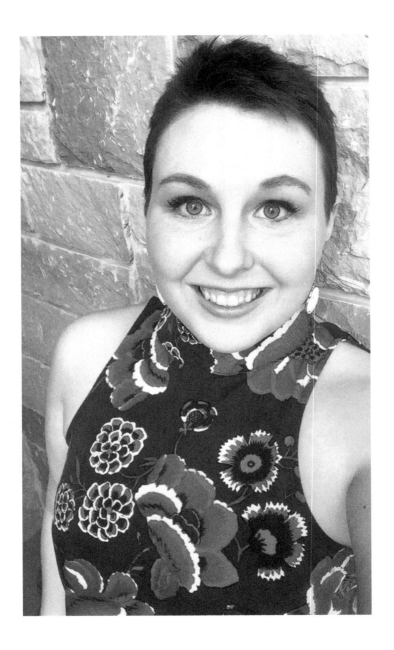

Kim's final thoughts:

> *"Finding out I had cancer was one of the toughest things to hear, but I think that day opened my eyes to living more purposefully. I now try to look for ways I can make a positive impact on others, and I have a better focus on my faith, family, and life goals."*

It seems like an oxymoron, but cancer does give gifts in the most unique and heartwarming way. Kim's both inspiring and strong. I'm looking forward to hearing how Kim's legislation unfolds.

PART FOUR:
THE FUTURE
OF PROTONS

THE FUTURE OF PROTONS: WHAT INNING ARE WE IN?

─────

I've always been active since I was a kid. I grew up playing sports, so sports analogies come natural to me. I played basketball, coached basketball, and was a cheerleader, too. I had a run with gymnastics which ended after a few years of miscoordination on the balance beam, but with a strong lesson from my coach and my mom to always get back up and on the beam.

Through all of the sports I played, baseball was my favorite. Back then, I was one of the first girls to play Little League with the boys' teams; girls didn't play much back then. I loved the length of the game starting before the sun sets and finishing under the evening lights. I remember the smell of spring and summer grass, the sound of crickets when I tried to catch balls in center field until I found my place with the boys in the infield defending third base. I loved the crack of the baseball bat, the sound it makes when the player connects with the ball. It means spring is here with new beginnings and the start of the baseball season.

As a baseball nut, I grew up a faithful Red Sox fan, so naturally I must really dislike the New York Yankees. It's part of growing up in Massachusetts—a rite of passage.

Fast forward, its 2021 and I feel like I'm in the third inning of my cancer journey, out of treatment now for three years. I'd like to get to the ninth inning as fast as I can but it doesn't work like that in cancer care.

As I learned more about proton radiation as part of my treatment plan, I couldn't help but wonder, what inning are we in with this modality?

So, using the analogy of baseball, I asked some of the radiation oncologists I interviewed:

What inning are we in with proton therapy?

I asked because on the one hand proton radiation has been approved by the FDA since 1988. It was suggested for use in treatment by a physicist who discovered how to harness its physical characteristics in the 1940s at Harvard University in the Harvard Cyclotron Laboratory. Massachusetts General Hospital, through the Harvard Cyclotron Laboratory, became the first in the world to use proton radiation for cancer care in 1956.

So, from this lens, it seems like we've played a lot of nine-inning baseball games in the field of proton radiation. But holistically, I wanted to get a sense of how far proton treatments have come to be able to understand the future potential of proton radiation in cancer care.

So, here's what the doctors had to say.

"I practice in Toronto, Canada. As of early-2021, there is not yet an active, definitive plan in any province to get shovels in the ground to build a proton therapy center to serve children and adults with cancer. This remains an unmet need for oncology in Canada, though cancer care agencies are trying to change this. Therefore, perhaps the national anthem has been sung, but the first pitch hasn't even been thrown. Or, as Canadians might say, the (hockey) puck hasn't dropped!"

—DEREK TSANG, MD, RADIATION ONCOLOGIST AT THE PRINCESS MARGARET CANCER CENTRE IN TORONTO, CANADA

"Wow, that's a good question. I'm a baseball person, too. I like the analogy. I'm going to go with a top of the fourth."

—DAVID A. BUSH, MD, PROFESSOR OF RADIATION MEDICINE, LOMA LINDA UNIVERSITY MEDICAL CENTER

I then asked about clinical trials and their impact on moving proton forward into other innings of the game.

"Yes, limiting access to clinical trials due to insurance coverage slows things down. *But a letter was issued by the National Cancer Institute (NCI) indicating certain randomized studies are necessary to determine whether proton therapy improves patient outcomes, and if so, by how much. The letter named specific trials and NCI encouraged insurance companies to cover treatment within these trials."*

—DAVID A. BUSH, MD, PROFESSOR OF RADIATION MEDICINE, LOMA LINDA UNIVERSITY MEDICAL CENTER

"Wow, I would say the first inning was the Harvard cyclotron in 1954. The second inning was Loma Linda with the world's first medical proton center using passive scatter. And the third inning is now introducing pencil beam scanning and a lot of the other things we normally do in X-ray therapy, we have a long, long, long way to go, though."

—CARL ROSSI, MD, RADIATION ONCOLOGIST, MEDICAL DIRECTOR, CALIFORNIA PROTONS CANCER THERAPY CENTER

"Even though 20 percent of cancer patients could benefit from proton therapy, less than 1 percent actually receive it. There is an enormous opportunity for this technology to expand. In fact, right here in the heart of Silicon Valley, we don't have proton therapy available locally."

—DEEPAK "DEE" KHUNTIA, MD, SENIOR VICE PRESIDENT, CHIEF MEDICAL OFFICER, VARIAN

"We're still in early innings in regard to the further elucidating and expanding the role of proton therapy globally. Broadly speaking, we are at an inflection point for the technology. Not in terms of its novelty but in terms of its growing applicability. Despite an expansion of proton therapy availability over the past decade, access issues remain from geographic, financial, and regulatory perspectives. Over the next five to ten years, we will see clinical use case scenarios continue to expand broadly across disease sites and the technology continue to advance. Coupling this with decreasing capital costs for equipment, we will likely see proton therapy transition from existing *in large-scale regional cancer programs to smaller-scale local programs."*

—GOPAL K. BAJAJ, MD, MBA RADIATION ONCOLOGIST, PRESIDENT, RADIATION ONCOLOGY ASSOCIATES, PC; VICE CHAIR OF THE GOVERNMENT RELATIONS COUNCIL FOR THE ASTRO BOARD OF DIRECTORS

"Great question! While protons have been around treating patients for decades, we are early in the game, just getting started at the top of the fourth inning. The technological innovations and clinical trials have expanded the benefits to more and more patients over the past few years. But we still have a long way to go to demonstrate the potential of protons and overcome barriers to access."

—MICHAEL J. EBLAN, MD, RADIATION ONCOLOGIST, RADIATION ONCOLOGY ASSOCIATES, PC

Finally, I asked: **What about proton radiation for breast cancer?**

"Decades ago, when we started treating partial breast cancer patients' insurance companies, of course, wouldn't pay for it. So, our hospital administration worked with us and we treated most of those patients at no cost at the beginning. Now today we can at least make an argument with insurance companies that now we have the data to say, 'see this is valid,' and it should be a covered treatment and for a number of insurance companies that has worked, not all of them, but a number of them it's worked."

—DAVID A. BUSH, MD, PROFESSOR OF RADIATION MEDICINE, LOMA LINDA UNIVERSITY MEDICAL CENTER

Cancer was like a curveball one minute, and a fastball the next. In late January of 2018, I was happily living my life, leaving a physical therapy appointment for my knee. I had too much wear and tear from playing sports as a kid, and I guess I was overdoing it in a boot camp class I was taking at the gym.

When I got the call from the breast imaging center to come back for more images, I didn't think twice about it. I literally thought I must have moved, and they needed more pictures. I even asked the person calling me if that's why I had to come back. She said she couldn't tell me why, but I needed to come back and preferably sooner than later. I should have picked up on that hint but feeling healthy and living life and being a rule follower, I called back and made an appointment for the next day.

When I reflect on my journey with protons, I'm in the early innings, yet it seems like the game's moved so fast. Although the treatment has been around since the 1940s, it still feels like we are in the third or fourth inning, with so much promise ahead. In baseball, it's hard to tell if the game's going to be fast or slow. Different variables like weather delays and competition play into the length of the game. I feel the same way about the different variables that play into protons' future.

So, what does the future look like for proton radiation?

"There [are] increasing amounts of data coming out and multiple adult cancers showing that the use of protons can reduce certain toxicities and in particular, the risk of radiation induced second cancers. So, if we can reduce that risk substantially, like a recent paper showed, this is

significant. There have been computer models predicting this for the last twenty years. If you can reduce secondary cancers and get the same cure rate, that's important.

Finally, like everything else in technology, the machines are getting less expensive, and therefore they're becoming a lot more financially viable and feasible for institutions to put in, they're getting smaller, too. So, this should have an impact on insurance approvals. This just mimics the history of X-ray therapy. You're going to see more and more centers opening, and protons will be much more widely distributed. People will have a greater amount of access to it than they did before."

—CARL ROSSI, MD, RADIATION ONCOLOGIST, MEDICAL DIRECTOR, CALIFORNIA PROTONS CANCER THERAPY CENTER

CONCLUSION

My goal for this book was to educate about proton radiation, what it is and what it isn't. The best way to know if it's right for a patient is to see a radiation oncologist who has access to both proton and photon radiation therapy.

Through our patient stories and physician input, it's evident proton radiation isn't experimental. Of the sixteen patients I interviewed, twelve were ultimately approved for treatment—a 75 percent approval rate. Two patients had self-funded plans, so their employers paid for treatments. Two patients were declined treatment, which is beyond unjust.

For many of us, protons taught us how to advocate. Cancer patients learn many lessons, and this is one of the best ones for me.

Through our patient stories, I hope these statistics and others in the book provide hope to patients who ask their doctor about a prescription for protons. It might just be the best prescription your doctor orders.

APPENDIX

INTRODUCTION

The Alliance for Proton Therapy Access. "Janelle Wright." Accessed July 1, 2021. https://allianceforprotontherapy.org/testimonial/janel-wright/.

ASTRO. "Prior Authorization Obstacles Unnecessarily Delay Patient Access to Cancer Treatments, Physician Survey Finds—American Society for Radiation Oncology (ASTRO)—American Society for Radiation Oncology (ASTRO)." April 25, 2019, https://www.astro.org/News-and-Publications/News-and-Media-Center/News-Releases/2019/Prior-authorization-obstacles-unnecessarily-delay.

CNBC. "Jury tells Aetna to Pay $25 Million to Late Cancer Patient's Family." November 11, 2018. https://www.cnbc.com/2018/11/11/jury-tells-aetna-to-pay-25-million-to-late-cancer-patients-family.html.

Drash, Wayne. "Judge Rips Insurance Company for 'Immoral, Barbaric' Cancer Denials." CNN, May 16, 2019. https://www.cnn.com/2019/05/16/health/judge-proton-beam-therapy-recusal-unitedhealthcare/index.html.

McCluskey, Priyanka Daya. "An Insurer Denied Her $95,000 Cancer Treatment. She's Fighting Back." *The Boston Globe*, May 4, 2019. https://www.bostonglobe.com/business/2019/05/04/promise-and-cost-clash-disputed-proton-cancer-treatment/MRX3NjsVc5RPtL-I7t9av8K/story.html.

PROTON BOB

Marckini, Robert J. *You Can Beat Prostate Cancer: And You Don't Need Surgery to Do It—New Edition*. Mattapoisett, MA: Robert J. Marckini, 2020.

Proton Bob. "About The BOB." Accessed February 21, 2021. https://protonbob.com/about-bob.

THE EVOLUTION OF RADIATION AND PROTON

American Cancer Society. "Do X-Rays and Gamma Rays Cause Cancer?" Accessed May 15, 2021. https://www.cancer.org/cancer/cancer-causes/radiation-exposure/x-rays-gamma-rays/do-xrays-and-gamma-rays-cause-cancer.html.

American Cancer Society. "Evolution of Cancer Treatments: Radiation." Accessed May 15, 2021. https://www.cancer.org/cancer/cancer-basics/history-of-cancer/cancer-treatment-radiation.html.

American Cancer Society. "Evolution of Cancer Treatments: Radiation." Accessed May 15, 2021. https://www.cancer.org/cancer/cancer-basics/history-of-cancer/cancer-treatment-radiation.html#:~:-text=Within%20months%2C%20systems%20were%20being,relatively%20low%2Dvoltage%20diagnostic%20machines.

Aronowitz, Jesse N. and Mark J. Rivard. "The Phylogeny of Permanent Prostate Brachytherapy." *Journal of Contemporary Brachytherapy* 2, no. 5 (June 28, 2013): pp. 89–92. https://doi.org/10.5114/jcb.2013.35562.

Carter, Devon. "Pencil Beam Proton Therapy: What to Know." MD Anderson Cancer Center. MD Anderson Cancer Center, August 7, 2019. https://www.mdanderson.org/cancerwise/pencil-beam-proton-therapy--what-to-know.h00-159305412.html.

CyberKnife. "How It Works." Accessed December 16, 2020. https://cyberknife.com/cyberknife-how-it-works/.

Giap, Huan, and Bosco Giap. "Historical perspective and evolution of charged particle beam therapy." "Translational Cancer Research." 2012;1(3):127–136. DOI: 10.3978/j.issn.2218-676X.2012.10.09.

Loma Linda University Cancer Center James M. Slater, MD Proton Treatment & Research Center. Accessed May 16, 2021. https://protons.com/.

Massachusetts General Hospital. "Proton Therapy." Accessed May 16, 2021. https://www.massgeneral.org/cancer-center/radiation-oncology/treatments-and-services/proton-therapy.

Memorial Sloan Kettering Cancer Center. "What Is IMRT?" Accessed May 19, 2021. https://www.mskcc.org/cancer-care/diagnosis-treatment/cancer-treatments/radiation-therapy/what-imrt.

National Cancer Institute. "Is Proton Therapy Safer than Traditional Radiation?" Accessed May 16, 2021. https://www.cancer.gov/

news-events/cancer-currents-blog/2020/proton-therapy-safety-versus-traditional-radiation.

National Cancer Institute. "NCI Dictionary of Cancer Terms." Accessed May 16, 2021. https://www.cancer.gov/publications/dictionaries/cancer-terms/def/photon-beam-radiation-therapy.

OncoLink Research Cancer Resources from OncoLink | Treatment. "Radiation Therapy: Which Type Is Right for Me?" Accessed May 16, 2021. https://www.oncolink.org/cancer-treatment/radiation/introduction-to-radiation-therapy/radiation-therapy-which-type-is-right-for-me.

Proton Therapy Today. "Why Is Proton Therapy the Preferable Option, and What is the Bragg Peak?" Accessed May 17, 2021. http://www.proton-therapy-today.com/what-is-proton-therapy/why-is-proton-therapy-a-preferable-option-and-what-is-the-bragg-peak/.

ACCESS TO PROTON THERAPY

Katipally, Rohan, BS and Deville Curtiland Jr., MD. "Health Disparities and Inequities in Radiation Therapy for Prostate Cancer." *Poster Abstract International Journal of Radiation Oncology, Biology, Physics*, June 2018, Volume 101, Issue 2.

Parikh-Patel, Arti et al., Supplement, E295. "A Population-Based Assessment of Proton Beam Therapy Utilization in California." *The American Journal of Managed Care* 26, no. 2 (May 2020). https://doi.org/10.37765/ajmc.2020.42398.

Sakurai, Hideyuki, Hitoshi Ishikawa, and Toshiyuki Okumura. "Proton Beam Therapy in Japan: Current and Future Status." OUP

Academic. Oxford University Press (October 11, 2016). https://academic.oup.com/jjco/article/46/10/885/2388083.

UMMCVideos. "Phoebe's Journey of Hope." June 22, 2016. Video, 6:152. https://www.youtube.com/watch?v=rU_ZyRh1aMM.

INSURANCE COVERAGE

American Medical Association. "2020 AMA Prior Authorization (PA) Physician Survey." Accessed March 11, 2021. https://www.ama-assn.org/system/files/2021-04/prior-authorization-survey.pdf.

American Medical Association. "2017 AMA Prior Authorization Physician Survey." February 2018. Accessed March 12, 2021. https://www.ama-assn.org/sites/ama-assn.org/files/corp/media-browser/public/arc/prior-auth-2017.pdf

ASCO. "CMS Urged to Reform Prior Authorization to Avoid Harm to Patients with Cancer." March 17, 2020. https://www.asco.org/practice-policy/policy-issues-statements/asco-in-action/cms-urged-reform-prior-authorization-avoid.

ASTRO. "Prior Authorization Obstacles Unnecessarily Delay Patient Access to Cancer Treatments, Physician Survey Finds—American Society for Radiation Oncology (ASTRO)—American Society for Radiation Oncology (ASTRO)." April 25, 2019. Accessed March 12, 2021. https://www.astro.org/News-and-Publications/News-and-Media-Center/News-Releases/2019/Prior-authorization-obstacles-unnecessarily-delay.

Boulay, Rick, MD. "Dear Insurance Doctor: You Are Not My Peer." KevinMD.com (blog). May 15, 2019. Accessed March 11,

2021. https://www.kevinmd.com/blog/2017/09/dear-insurance-doctor-not-peer.html.

HCAA Videos. "HCAA's Self-Funding Primer." March 26, 2017. Video, 2:48. https://youtu.be/3jZhFXJYSUU.

Maryland Proton Treatment Center. Accessed March 11, 2021. https://mdproton.com/.

Murphy, Tom. "Health Claim Rejected? Some Steps to Appeal a Denial." AP NEWS Associated Press, May 8, 2019. https://apnews.com/article/health-50f61742999c457a9f3e35c9336606b8.

New York Proton Center. "Getting Proton Therapy Covered By Insurance." Accessed March 11, 2021. https://www.nyproton.com/insurance/.

Robeznieks, Andis. "Inside Cleveland Clinic's $10 Million Prior Authorization Price Tag." *AMA*, November 16, 2018. https://www.ama-assn.org/practice-management/sustainability/inside-cleveland-clinic-s-10-million-prior-authorization-price.

HOW DOES THE VARIAN PROTON MACHINE WORK?

Mehta, Minesh. "Proton Therapy Predictions for the Next Decade." *Imaging Technology News*, July 7, 2020. https://www.itnonline.com/article/proton-therapy-predictions-next-decade.

Varian. Accessed June 28, 2021. https://www.varian.com/.

COST SAVINGS, HIGHER QUALITY OF CARE
THE RADIATION ONCOLOGY (RO) ALTERNATIVE
PAYMENT MODEL (APM)

AHA. American Hospital Association to Seema Verna, Washington, DC, September 16, 2019. "Radiation Oncology APM Comment-Letter." https://www.aha.org/system/files/media/file/2019/09/Radiation-Oncology_APM-Comment-

ASTRO. American Society for Radiation Oncologists to Seema Verna, Washington, DC, September 16, 2019. "Medicare Program; Specialty Care Models to Improve Quality of Care and Reduce Expenditures."

https://www.astro.org/ASTRO/media/ASTRO/Daily%20Practice/PDFs/ASTRO-ROModelFinalCommentLetter.pdf

CMS. "Fact Sheet Radiation Oncology (RO) Model Fact Sheet." Accessed May 30, 2021. https://www.cms.gov/newsroom/fact-sheets/radiation-oncology-ro-model-fact-sheet#_ftn1.

Guideway Care. "RO-APM: What Providers Need to Know About the New Model." October 26, 2020. https://guidewaycare.com/ro-apm-what-providers-need-to-know/.

Innovation.cms.gov. "United States Department of Health and Human Services Report to Congress: Episodic Alternative Payment Model for Radiation Therapy Services." Department of Health and Human Services, November 2017. Accessed December 5, 2020. https://innovation.cms.gov/files/reports/radiationtherapy-apm-rtc.pdf.

Medicare. "What's Medicare?" Accessed June 28, 2021. https://www.medicare.gov/what-medicare-covers/your-medicare-coverage-choices/whats-medicare.

National Institutes of Health. United States Department of Health and Human Services. "Cancer Costs Projected to Reach at Least $158 Billion in 2020." September 25, 2015. https://www.nih.gov/news-events/news-releases/cancer-costs-projected-reach-least-158-billion-2020.

CLINICAL TRIALS

Bauman, Brian MD. "Locally Advanced Cancer: Proton vs Photon Therapy." Study presented at the Annual Meeting of the American Society for Clinical Oncology ASCO, Chicago, IL, June 2019. https://ascopost.com/videos/2019-asco-annual-meeting/brian-baumann-on-proton-vs-photon-therapy-in-locally-advanced-cancer/.

FDA United States Food and Drug Administration. "What Are the Different Types of Clinical Research?" Accessed June 28, 2021. https://www.fda.gov/patients/clinical-trials-what-patients-need-know/what-are-different-types-clinical-research.

Fuller, Felicia. "Imperialcrs.com." *Imperialcrs.com* (blog). Imperial Research Clinical Services, October 29, 2015. https://www.imperialcrs.com/blog/2015/10/29/25-reasons-people-arent-enrolling-in-your-clinical-trial/. Accessed May 31, 2021.

National Cancer Institute. "Clinical Trials Information for Patients and Caregivers." Accessed June 28, 2021. https://www.cancer.gov/about-cancer/treatment/clinical-trials.

Tekton Research. "Phases of Clinical Trials." Provided by National Comprehensive Cancer Network, July 28, 2020. https://tekton-research.com/phases-of-clinical-trials/.

THE PATIENT EXPERIENCE

Noseworthy, John. "The Future of Care—Preserving the Patient–Physician Relationship: NEJM." New England Journal of Medicine, December 5, 2019. https://www.nejm.org/doi/full/10.1056/NEJMsr1912662.

Wolf, Jason A. "*A Global Inquiry on Excellence in the Diagnostic Journey: The Power of Human Experience in Healthcare.*" The Beryl Institute PX White Papers, 2020, https://www.theberylinstitute.org/store/download.aspx?id=122D0D7B-B8AC-4B07-9102-6CB76EF5A34A.

PROTONS AND BREAST CANCER

American Cancer Society. "Radiation for Breast Cancer." Accessed March 14, 2021. https://www.cancer.org/cancer/breast-cancer/treatment/radiation-for-breast-cancer.html.

California Protons. "Proton Therapy for Breast Cancer—CA Protons Tumor Treatment." November 5, 2020. https://www.californiaprotons.com/breast-cancer/.

Lorenzen, E. Laugaard, J. Christian, Rehammar, M. B .Jensen et al. "Radiation-induced risk of ischemic heart disease following breast cancer radiotherapy in Denmark." 1977–2005, Radiotherapy and Oncology. https://doi.org/10.1016/j.radonc.2020.08.007.

MD Anderson Cancer Center. "Breast Cancer." Accessed March 14, 2021. https://www.mdanderson.org/patients-family/diagnosis-treatment/care-centers-clinics/proton-therapy-center/conditions-we-treat/breast-cancer.html.

Oncotypeiq. "About the Oncotype DX Breast Recurrence Score® Test: Oncotype IQ® Canada." Accessed March 20, 2021. https://www.oncotypeiq.com/en-CA/breast-cancer/patients-and-caregivers/stage-i-iiia-invasive/about-the-test.

Oncotypeiq. "Node-Positive Clinical Evidence: Oncotype DX® Test: Oncotype IQ® Canada." Accessed March 20, 2021. https://www.oncotypeiq.com/en-CA/breast-cancer/healthcare-professionals/oncotype-dx-breast-recurrence-score/node-positive-clinical-evidence.

Stony Brook Cancer Center. "Respiratory Gating and Deep Inspiration Breath Hold (DIBH)." Accessed March 20, 2021. https://cancer.stonybrookmedicine.edu/diagnosis-treatment/radiation-oncology/treatment-technology/respiratory-gating#:~:text=Respiratory%20Deep%20Inspiration%20Breath,cycle%20of%20inspiration%20and%20expiration.

UF Health Proton Therapy Institute. "Effective Breast Cancer Treatment." Accessed March 21, 2021. https://www.floridaproton.org/ppc/breast-cancer-free.

MARIAM'S STORY

Ambry Genetics, A Konica Minolta Company. "Understanding your TP53 Genetic Test Result." Accessed January 27, 2021. https://www.ambrygen.com/material/oncology/understanding-your-results/tp53/1039.

American Cancer Society. "Second Cancers Related to Treatment." Accessed January 28, 2021. https://www.cancer.org/treatment/treatments-and-side-effects/physical-side-effects/second-cancers-in-adults.html

BreastCancer.org. "Stage 3 (III) A, B and C." Accessed January 28th, 2021. https://www.nationalbreastcancer.org/breast-cancer-stage-3.

Healthline. "Chemotherapy and Targeted Therapy for HER2-Positive Breast Cancer." Accessed January 25, 2021. https://www.healthline.com/health/breast-cancer/chemotherapy-for-her2-positive-breast-cancer#targeted-therapy.

KGTV. "Young Cancer Survivor Fights for Patient Rights after Insurance Denies Proton Therapy." June 5, 2018. https://www.10news.com/news/young-cancer-survivor-fights-for-patient-rights-after-insurance-denies-proton-therapy.

Mayo Clinic. "HER-positive Breast Cancer." Accessed January 25, 2021. https://www.mayoclinic.org/breast-cancer/expert-answers/faq-20058066.

Mayo Clinic. "Positron Emission Tomography." Accessed January 29, 2021. https://www.mayoclinic.org/tests-procedures/pet-scan/about/pac-20385078.

O'Brien, Jack. "UnitedHealth Delivers Strong Q4 Earnings to End 2018." *HealthLeaders Media*, January 15, 2019. https://www.healthleadersmedia.com/finance/unitedhealth-delivers-strong-q4-earnings-end-2018.

OncoLink. "Pictorial Overview of the Proton Therapy Treatment Process." Accessed January 28, 2021. https://es.oncolink.org/tratamiento-del-cancer/terapia-con-proton/resumen/pictorial-overview-of-the-proton-therapy-treatment-process.

Tariq, Mariam. "Insurance Denied When Most Needed: Healing a Broken Health-Care System by Holding Insurers Accountable." *Santa Barbara Independent*, March 30, 2019. https://www.independent.com/2019/03/30/insurance-denied-when-most-needed/.

Yu, Nathan Y. et al. "The Insurance Approval Process for Proton Beam Therapy Must Change: Prior Authorization Is Crippling Access to Appropriate Health Care." *International Journal of Radiation Oncology, Biology, Physics*, 104, no. 4 (2019): pp. 737–739, https://doi.org/10.1016/j.ijrobp.2019.04.007.

PROTONS & HEAD & NECK CANCER

HEAD COACH RON RIVERA THE WASHINGTON FOOTBALL TEAM

ASTRO. "Prior Authorization Obstacles Unnecessarily Delay Patient Access to Cancer Treatments, Physician Survey Finds" April 25, 2019. https://www.astro.org/News-and-Publications/News-and-Media-Center/News-Releases/2019/Prior-authorization-obstacles-unnecessarily-delay.

Good Morning America (GMA). "Washington Football Team Head Coach Talks Cancer Battle." October 5, 2020. Video, 5:02. https://www.youtube.com/watch?v=9vqEkn7Ttqk.

Hackett, Mallory. "CMS Receives Payer Pushback on Final Interoperability and Prior Authorization Rule." *Healthcare Finance*

News, January 19, 2021. https://www.healthcarefinancenews.com/news/cms-receives-payer-pushback-final-interoperability-and-prior-authorization-rule.

Keim, John. "Washington Coach Ron Rivera Cheered at Hospital as Cancer Treatments Finish." *ESPN*. ESPN Internet Ventures, October 26, 2020. https://www.espn.com/nfl/story/_/id/30197801/washington-coach-ron-rivera-cheered-hospital-cancer-treatments-finish. Accessed January, February 14, 2021.

MGMA. "MGMA Statement on CMS Interoperability and Prior Authorization Final Rule." January 15, 2021. https://www.mgma.com/advocacy/advocacy-statements-letters/advocacy-statements/mgma-statement-on-cms-interoperability-and-prior-a.

Richard, Julie. "Pre-Treatment Dental Issues." The Oral Cancer Foundation (An MD Anderson Perspective). Accessed February 14, 2021. https://oralcancerfoundation.org/dental/pre-treatment-dental-issues/.

Stempniak, Marty. "Providers and Payers Unite in Blasting 'Hastily Constructed' CMS Final Rule to Simplify Prior Authorization." *Radiology Business*, April 2, 2021. https://www.radiologybusiness.com/topics/imaging-informatics/cms-final-rule-simplify-prior-authorization.

Stanford Health Care. "Metastatic Squamous Neck Cancer with Occult Primary." Accessed February 14, 2021. https://stanfordhealthcare.org/medical-conditions/cancer/metastatic-squamous-neck-cancer.html

Tikkanen, Roosa and Melinda K Abrams. "United States Health Care from a Global Perspective, 2019: Higher Spending, Worse

Outcomes?" *Commonwealth Fund*, January 30, 2020. https://
www.commonwealthfund.org/publications/issue-briefs/2020/jan/
us-health-care-global-perspective-2019?gclid=CjwKCAiAsaOB-
BhA4EiwAoo_AnBwffa8H6PVxYi-kq-caCYiBNyQfaRbuagNd9zY-
FXvfBJoZlidHC2RoCIesQAvD_BwE.

BRIAN'S STORY

AAFP. "Independent Physicians Associations, (Ipa)." Accessed
January 30, 2021. https://www.aafp.org/about/policies/all/inde-
pendent-physician-associations.html

Blanchard, Pierre et al. "Intensity-Modulated Proton Beam Therapy (IMPT) versus Intensity-Modulated Photon Therapy (IMRT)
for Patients with Oropharynx Cancer—A Case Matched Analysis." Radiotherapy and oncology: journal of the European Society
for Therapeutic Radiology and Oncology (United States National
Library of Medicine), accessed February 8, 2021. https://pubmed.
ncbi.nlm.nih.gov/27342249/.

California Protons Therapy Center. " Our Physicians." Accessed
January 30, 2021. https://www.californiaprotons.com/

Cancer.Net. "Head and Neck Cancer." June 17, 2014. https://www.
cancer.net/cancer-types/head-and-neck-cancer.

Meridian Allenpress. "Trends and Disparities of Proton Therapy
Use among Patients with Head and Neck Cancer: Analysis from
the National Cancer Database (2005-14)." April 22, 2019. https://
meridian.allenpress.com/theijpt/article/5/4/1/432758/Trends-and-
Disparities-of-Proton-Therapy-Use-among.

PROTON & PROSTATE CANCER

JOHN'S STORY

American Cancer Society. "Prostate Cancer Risk Factors." Accessed February 20, 2021. https://www.cancer.org/cancer/prostate-cancer/causes-risks-prevention/risk-factors.html.

American Cancer Society. "Tests to Diagnose and Stage Prostate Cancer." Accessed February 20, 2021. https://www.cancer.org/cancer/prostate-cancer/detection-diagnosis-staging/how-diagnosed.html.

Marckini, Robert J. *You Can Beat Prostate Cancer: And You Don't Need Surgery to Do It—New Edition.* Mattapoisett, MA: Robert J. Marckini, 2020.

Mayo Clinic. "Prostate Brachytherapy." March 10, 2020. https://www.mayoclinic.org/tests-procedures/prostate-brachytherapy/about/pac-20384949.

National Cancer Institute. "NCI Dictionary of Cancer Terms." Accessed June 29, 2021. https://www.cancer.gov/publications/dictionaries/cancer-terms/def/ajcc-staging-system.

NCCN. "Patient and Caregiver Resources." Accessed February 20, 2021. https://www.nccn.org/patients/.

JIM'S STORY

American Cancer Society. "Baltimore Hope Lodge Facilities: Housing Assistance For Cancer Patients." Accessed February 21, 2021. https://www.cancer.org/treatment/support-programs-and-services/patient-lodging/hope-lodge/baltimore/about-our-facility.html.

American Cancer Society. "Tests to Diagnose and Stage Prostate Cancer." Accessed February 21, 2021. https://www.cancer.org/cancer/prostate-cancer/detection-diagnosis-staging/how-diagnosed.html.

Cancer.net. "Prostate Cancer—Stages and Grades." Accessed January 27, 2021. https://www.cancer.net/cancer-types/prostate-cancer/stages-and-grades.

Hyun, Jae Saog. "Prostate Cancer and Sexual Function." *The World Journal of Men's Health.* V. 30 (2) (Aug 2012): 99–107

Mayo Clinic. "PSA Test." May 4, 2019. https://www.mayoclinic.org/tests-procedures/psa-test/about/pac-20384731.

Murphy, Tom. "Health Claim Rejected? Some Steps to Appeal a Denial." *AP NEWS,* May 8, 2019. https://apnews.com/article/50f-61742999c457a9f3e35c9336606b8.

National Nurses United. "60–80% Of Insurance Denials Overturned or Reversed When Taken to Independent Medical Review—New Data." California Nurses Association, February 28, 2018. https://www.nationalnursesunited.org/press/60-80-insurance-denials-overturned-or-reversed-when-taken-independent-medical-review-new-data.

DAN'S STORY

FDA. "FDA Approves First PSMA-Targeted PET Imaging Drug for Men with Prostate Cancer." December 1, 2020. https://www.fda.gov/news-events/press-announcements/fda-approves-first-psma-targeted-pet-imaging-drug-men-prostate-cancer.

GE Healthcare. "Whole-Body Diffusion for Evaluation of Metastatic Lesions." Accessed March 4, 2021, https://www.gehealthcare.com/article/whole-body-diffusion-mri-for-the-evaluation-of-metastatic-lesions.

Rosenkrantz, AB, J. Hemingway, Hughes DR et al. "Evolving use of Prebiopsy Prostate Magnetic Resonance Imaging in the Medicare Population." *The Journal of Urology*, 2018;200:89–94.

PROTONS & PEDIATRIC BRAIN CANCER

NIKKI'S STORY

St. Jude Children's Hospital. "Medulloblastoma." Accessed February 13, 2021. https://www.stjude.org/disease/medulloblastoma.html

GRACE'S STORY

ABTA. "Proton Therapy." accessed January 24, 2021. https://www.abta.org/publications/proton-therapy/.

Alliance for Proton Therapy Access. "Our Stories." Accessed January 24, 2021. https://allianceforprotontherapy.org/

American Childhood Cancer Organization. "Gold Ribbon Hero Grace." Accessed January 23, 2021. https://www.acco.org/blog/grh-grace-at-sotu-2019/.

Brinley, Maryann. "Saving Grace." RWJBarnabas Health Rutgers Cancer Institute of New Jersey. Accessed January 31, 2021. Saving Grace | Rutgers Cancer Institute of New Jersey (cinj.org).

Fox News. "10-Year-Old Cancer Survivor Describes Attending the SOTU." Video, 4:01. https://www.youtube.com/watch?v=OOsk-NvV6moc.

Gottheimer.house.gov. "Gottheimer Leading Bipartisan Legislation to Boost Investment in Pediatric Cancer Research to Find More Cures, Save Lives." United States Representative Josh Gottheimer, May 25, 2021. https://gottheimer.house.gov/news/documentsingle.aspx?DocumentID=2531

RWJ Barnabas Health Rutgers Cancer Institute of New Jersey, Let's Beat Cancer Together. "Saving Grace." Video, 3:36. https://youtu.be/Yhu6ivcfJeU.

St. Jude's Children's Hospital. "Germ Cell Tumors (Brain)." Accessed January 23, 2021. https://www.stjude.org/disease/germ-cell-tumors-brain.html.

The Valerie Fund, Accessed January 24, 2021. https://www.thevaleriefund.org/.

WITH Grace Initiative. Accessed January 24, 2021. https://www.withgraceinitiative.org/

PROTONS & LYMPHOMA

KEELIN'S STORY

American Cancer Society. "Hodgkin Lymphoma Stages: Hodgkin Disease Stages." Accessed February 26, 2021. https://www.cancer.org/cancer/hodgkin-lymphoma/detection-diagnosis-staging/staging.html.

Cancer.net. "Lymphoma—Hodgkin—Statistics." Accessed January 29, 2021. https://www.cancer.net/cancer-types/lymphoma-hodgkin/statistics.

Dana-Farber Cancer Institute. "Amy Gross, How to Manage Fear of Cancer Recurrence." May 3, 2010. Video, 6:08. https://www.youtube.com/watch?v=xlYUytWtlK8.

PROTONS & THYMUS CANCER

EVA'S STORY

American Cancer Society. "What is Thymus Cancer? "Accessed February 3, 2021. www.cancer.org

CDC. "New ICD-10-CM code for the 2019 Novel Coronavirus (COVID-19). April 1, 2020. Effective: March 18, 2020." Accessed February 2, 2021. https://www.cdc.gov/nchs/data/icd/Announcement-New-ICD-code-for-coronavirus-3-18-2020.pdf

Cedars Sinai. "Thymoma." Accessed January 31st, 2021. https://www.cedars-sinai.org/health-library/diseases-and-conditions/t/thymoma.html.

Frankenfield, Jake. "Which Industry Spends the Most on Lobbying?" *Investopedia*, August 28, 2020. https://www.investopedia.com/investing/which-industry-spends-most-lobbying-antm-so/#:~:-text=Spending%20%244.45%20billion%20over%20the,other%20industries%20in%20lobbying%20spending.

Gostin, Lawrence J.D. L.D. D. "The Formulation of Health Policy by the Three Branches of Government." *Society's Choices: Social and Ethical Decision Making in Biomedicine. United States National Library of Medicine*, January 1, 1995. https://www.ncbi.nlm.nih.gov/books/NBK231979/.

Medline Plus. "Pericardial Disorders." Accessed January 31, 2021. https://medlineplus.gov/pericardialdisorders.html

O'Connor, Matt. "Prior Authorization Is Hurting Patients and Radiation Oncologists, Survey Finds." *Health Imaging*, April 26, 2019. https://www.healthimaging.com/topics/oncology-imaging/prior-authorization-hurting-patients-radiation-oncologists.

ABOUT ADVOCACY

Patient Advocate Foundation. Accessed February 6, 2021. https://www.patientadvocate.org/

CATHLEEN'S STORY OF ADENOID CYSTIC CARCINOMA, ADVOCACY & FAITH IN GOD

Cancer.Net. "Adenoid Cystic Carcinoma: Statistics." Accessed February 6, 2021. https://www.cancer.net/cancer-types/adenoid-cystic-carcinoma/statistics

Kneler, Ph.D., Andrew W. et al. "Cancer: Religion and Spirituality." *Stanford Medicine, Surviving Cancer.* Accessed June 1, 2021. https://med.stanford.edu/survivingcancer/cancer-sources-of-support/cancer-religion-spirituality-help.html.

MD Anderson Cancer Center. "About Dr. Hanna." Accessed February 6, 2021. https://faculty.mdanderson.org/profiles/ehab_y_hanna.html#:~:text=Ehab%20Hanna%2C%20M.D.%2C%20FACS%2C-Cancer%20Center%20in%20Houston%2C%20Texas.

Visiontree Global Health Cloud. "About Us." Accessed February 6, 2021. https://www.visiontree.com/about-us/.

KATE'S STORY & YOUR LEGAL RIGHTS

Callahan & Blaine. "Rich Collins & Proton Beam Therapy Insurance Denials." March 3, 2021. https://litigation-update.com/proton-beam-therapy-pbt-insurance-denials/.

Dana-Faber. Accessed June 17, 2021. https://www.dana-farber.org/newsroom/news-releases/2020/newsweek-names-dana-farber--3-in-the-world-for-cancer/.

Drash, Wayne. "When Insurance Wouldn't Pay, Parents Funded Cancer Patient's $95,000 Lifesaving Treatment." CNN, August 17, 2018. https://www.cnn.com/2018/08/15/health/cancer-survivor-insurance-denial-battle/index.html.

Grzincic, Barbara. "IN BRIEF: UnitedHealthcare Can't Zap Cancer Survivors' Lawsuit over Proton Therapy." Reuters, March 9, 2021. https://www.reuters.com/article/united-proton-lawsuit/in-brief-unitedhealthcare-cant-zap-cancer-survivors-lawsuit-over-proton-therapy-idUSL1N2L707U.

Kantor & Kantor LLP. "Cancer Survivor Kate Weissman Files Spearheading Class Action Lawsuit to Expose UnitedHealthcare's Pursuit of Profits over Patient Protection and Care." March 19, 2019.

https://www.californiainsurancelawyerblog.com/cancer-survivor-kate-weissman-files-spearheading-class-action-lawsuit-to-expose-unitedhealthcares-pursuit-of-profits-over-patient-protection-and-care/

Kolakowski, Mark. "10 Biggest Healthcare Companies." *Investopedia*, July 30, 2020. https://www.investopedia.com/articles/markets/030916/worlds-top-10-health-care-companies-unh-mdt.asp

McCluskey, Priyanka Daya. "An Insurer Denied Her $95,000 Cancer Treatment. She's Fighting Back." *The Boston Globe*, May 4, 2019. https://www.bostonglobe.com/business/2019/05/04/promise-and-cost-clash-disputed-proton-cancer-treatment/MRX3NjsVc5RPtL-I7t9av8K/story.html.

Schlein, Zach. "Cancer-Survivor Judge Steps Down From Case Over Insurer's Coverage Denial." *ThinkAdvisor*, April 30, 2019. https://www.thinkadvisor.com/2019/04/30/cancer-survivor-judge-steps-down-from-case-over-insurers-barbaric-denial-of-treatment-415-330733/.

KIM'S STORY

Cancer.Net. "Lymphoma—Non-Hodgkin—Stages." January 28, 2020. https://www.cancer.net/cancer-types/lymphoma-non-hodgkin/stages.

Cancer Treatment Centers of America. "About Hodgkin Lymphoma: Information, Facts & Overview." November 4, 2020. https://www.cancercenter.com/cancer-types/hodgkin-lymphoma/about.

Cancer Treatment Centers of America. "Difference between Blood Cancers: Leukemia & Lymphoma." July 14, 2020. https://www.cancercenter.com/community/blog/2018/05/whats-the-difference-blood-cancers-leukemia-lymphoma-and-multiple-myeloma.

EviCore. "About EviCore." Accessed February 22, 2021. https://www.evicore.com/about.

THE FUTURE OF PROTONS WHAT INNING ARE WE IN?

Massachusetts General Hospital. "Proton Therapy." Accessed February 27, 2021. https://www.massgeneral.org/cancer-center/radiation-oncology/treatments-and-services/proton-therapy.

FDA. Center for Biologics Evaluation and Research. "Emergency Use Authorization for Vaccines Explained." Accessed June 20, 2021. https://www.fda.gov/vaccines-blood-biologics/vaccines/emergency-use-authorization-vaccines-explained.

National Cancer Institute. "Cancer Statistics." Accessed June 21, 2021. https://www.cancer.gov/about-cancer/understanding/statistics.

PATIENT RESOURCES

———

In this section you'll find resources that may be helpful to consider during your cancer journey with protons.

INSURANCE

- Ask about the cost of proton and photon treatment in the first consultation if you are considering either treatment. At the Maryland Proton Treatment Center, when I was treated, the cost of both was the same.
- Ask about the insurance process at the time of the first consult.
- Understand many times the first and second prior-authorization request for payment to insurance is denied. With your doctor's advice, appeal the first and second denials, and keep fighting for insurance coverage if the doctor feels you can safely do so.
- Consider other proton centers that might offer different pricing structures for your proton treatment plan.
- Go online and get a copy of your insurance policy. Read what is covered and what isn't covered.
- Find out if your insurance is self-funded. If it is, this means your company or organization could ultimately

pay for your treatment, like Cathleen McBurney and Keelin McGee's stories.

- Call the pre-authorization coordinator at the cancer center or your doctor and ask for a copy of the denial letter. Save the letter(s).
- Contact insurance and talk to them about your denial and get their responses in writing if possible.
- If your claim is denied on the first and second try, find out the name and medical specialty of the doctor at the insurance company that denied your claim. Ask, is this doctor a radiation oncologist that denied my case?
- Keep track of how many denials and appeals have been made on your behalf.
- Ask your doctor for a copy of your Letter of Medical Necessity (LMN) or comparative plan.

CLINICAL TRIALS

All clinical trials in the United States are listed at www.clinicaltrials.gov.

Here's a list of things to consider when deciding on whether to join a trial or not:

- How long is the trial? Although anyone can drop out of a trial at any time, this should be discussed with the patient who's enrolled.
- How many more office visits will be required on top of regular follow up appointments?
- Will it cost more money in travel, or will you need lodging to enter a trial that isn't close to home?
- Your data will be protected and not disclosed.

- Discuss your decision with friends, family, your doctor, and maybe other people who have been through a clinical trial before.
- Think about the mental health implications of more doctor visits. Will this affect your ability to move forward after cancer treatment?

MENTAL HEALTH CONSIDERATIONS

- Being diagnosed with cancer is scary. At diagnosis, during and especially in after care, it can be stressful and ridden with anxiety. I met with a therapist a few times during diagnosis, treatment, and thereafter. It was incredibly helpful.
- Ask your doctor for a reference to a mental health specialist.
- Consider talking to a licensed clinical social worker (LCSW) or other mental health specialist that is credentialed in oncology care.
- Find a therapist near you at https://www.psychologytoday.com/us/therapists/cancer.
- Journal your thoughts and bring them to your therapist.
- Look back on the progress you've made since diagnosis.

SLEEP DISRUPTIONS

- Talk to your doctor if you feel fatigued. Napping may impact the ability to sleep through the night, which could impact your healing. I know this happened to me.
- Seek a therapist that can help with diagnosing you for clinical insomnia. I was diagnosed with clinical insomnia eighteen months after treatment. I entered a Cognitive Behavior Therapy for Insomnia (CBTI) program and my

insomnia was cured for the most part. This program isn't easy but is worth it if you do the work.

- You can find several resources on CBTI and other sleep concerns at the National Sleep Foundation; https://www.sleepfoundation.org/insomnia/treatment/cognitive-behavioral-therapy-insomnia

NUTRITION

- Ask your doctor what's best for nutrition.
- Stay hydrated but be careful not to overhydrate.
- Work with a nutritionist, one who has a specialty in oncology nutrition. Many cancer centers offer this type of service at the center.

SKIN CARE

- Ask your doctor about lotions for your skin if the lotions provided don't help. With my doctor's approval, I used Spectrum Coconut Oil found at Whole Foods and on Amazon. It helped me so much!

ACKNOWLEDGMENTS

———

There are simply not enough words to thank everyone who helped me create this book, starting with every patient and family I interviewed. I felt bad asking you to retell your stories, yet I know we all want to share our stories so we can educate about protons and help others. I'm forever grateful.

To the physicians I interviewed, at night or over the weekend during their busy days in their clinics, thank you. I also appreciate your help in getting your input accurately captured. Your trust in me to tell the story of protons from the lenses of science, physics, advocacy, and your clinical experience brought credibility to the field of proton radiation for new patients. Special thanks to Dr. Eblan and Dr Bajaj who read a few chapters for clinical accuracy and thank you to Dr. Chhabra who helped me firm up the subtitle. I appreciate you all so much.

Before this book was published, I helped one friend learn more about protons and she just started treatment this week. Dr. Eblan, Dr. Chhabra, and Dr. Choi, thank you for offering to talk to her, and thank you for helping me help her. I'm so grateful.

To my medical team, Dr. Eblan, Dr. Edmiston, Dr. Rad, and Dr. Harnden, thank you for healing me through your expertise and compassion. I can't thank you enough.

To everyone who bought a pre-sale copy of my book, your support means so much, thank you.

Joanne Haight, Anne Durgin, Robin Durgin-King, Mark Brahms, Katie Maloney, Molly Maloney, Patrick Maloney, Megan Maloney, Craig Mason, Heidi Day, Brian Berry, Anne Marie Wemmlinger, Heleen Westerhuijs, Louise Loyst, Cathy King, John Caslione, Nicole Cable-Bailey, Tim Hill, Maureen Dalbec, Maureen DiMestico, Noreen Richards, Susan Curtin, Lisa Jessick, Patricia Kehoe, Carlo Mahfouz, Eric Koester, Grant DeMola Irena Djordjevic Behery, Nadine Kwebetchou, Gail Sharpe, Jeff Evans, Kate Emily Weissman, Eva Tai, Nancy Bowles, Allison Valley, Cathleen C McBurney, Keelin McGee, Kathrin Hashemi, Tammy Douglas McPhee, Kira Brunjes, Helen Su, Ann Rhie Kubera, Rita & Mark Kearns, Michele Boshar, Patrick & Denise Byrne, Kelli Bland, Falisha Alie, Kevin Blafkin, Peter Crews, Gloria Ayure, Nadya Mhmd, Rajeswari Ramanan, Rich Collins, Aubrey Reichard-Eline, Keith Olson, Cameron& Ellie Marlow, Sandra Carrie, Paige Duke Debra Durgin-Glenn, Dave O'Connor, George & Michelle Nash, Nura Mendez, Elaine Czarnecki, Pam Wesemann, Dalia Hidayat, Randy Novia, Janie Haeger, Jan Antons, Frank Rosenthal, lyse Veron, Stacia Hepburn, Noel Sweeney, Sarah Drijfhout, Aaron Alberico, Lisa Dahl, Tegest H. Dirasse, Tracey Leacoma, Ann Gleason, Nancy Terry, Tom & JoJo Maloney.

To my husband Patrick, who hasn't seen much of me since I started writing this book in October of 2020, you are my rock. You supported me through breast cancer, and the challenges thereafter with rib fractures and Tamoxifen. I might have worn out our vows "in sickness and in health." I love you.

To my mom, sister, dad, four stepdaughters, son-in-law, granddaughter, two pups Stewie and Stella, and all my dear friends and family—I'm so lucky to be in your village. Mom, I can't thank you enough for your texts, cards, constant support, and your help in buying books for so many people. My dad, "I can't wait to read your book." To my sister, you are my angel, always there for me and... The Network. I love you.

Thank you Eric Koester for this experience to create! Finally, to my editing and publishing team, Tricia Gamma, Vivian Rose, Christy Mossburg, Mackenzie Joyce, and Brian Bies, thank you for your support.

Joanne, thank you for inspiring me through the song, "This Little Light of Mine."

I want my light to shine through to help others for years to come. Amen.

Made in United States
North Haven, CT
20 November 2021

11317929R00192